Pharma, Exploitation, and Poor Communities

Revolutionary Bioethics

Series Editor: Rachel Haliburton, University of Sudbury

Revolutionary Bioethics is a new series composed of scholarly monographs and edited collections organized around specific topics that explore bioethical theory and practice through the frameworks provided by feminist ethics, narrative ethics, and virtue ethics, challenging the assumptions of mainstream bioethics in the process. Contemporary mainstream bioethics has become ideological and repetitive, a defender of activities that bioethics was originally created to critique, and an apologist for unethical practices and policies in medicine that it once saw itself as fighting against. Taking its title from recent work being done on MacIntyre's neo-Aristotelian ethics, Revolutionary Bioethics is organized around the idea that bioethics needs to reform both its theory and practice, and its goal is to begin the conversation about what a transformed bioethics—one that is unafraid to explore new theoretical approaches, and to examine and critique current bioethical practices—might look like.

Titles in the Series

Pharma, Exploitation, and Poor Communities: Rethinking the Ethics of Global Research through Fair Play, by Felicitas Sofia Holzer

Bioethical Responsibilities in Twenty-First Century Crises, edited by Elizabeth Lanphier and Larry R. Churchill

Redescribing Bioethics: How the Field Constructs Its Argument, by Tod S. Chambers

Righting Health Policy: Bioethics, Political Philosophy, and the Normative Justification of Health Law and Policy, by D. Robert MacDougall

Caregiving, Carebots, and Contagion, by Michael C. Brannigan

Engineering Perfection: Solidarity, Disability, and Well-being, by Elyse Purcell

Physician-Assisted Suicide and Euthanasia: Before, During, and After the Third Reich, edited by Sheldon Rubenfeld and Daniel P. Sulmasy, with Astrid Ley

Pharma, Exploitation, and Poor Communities

Rethinking the Ethics of Global Research through Fair Play

Felicitas Sofia Holzer

BLOOMSBURY ACADEMIC
NEW YORK • LONDON • OXFORD • NEW DELHI • SYDNEY

BLOOMSBURY ACADEMIC
Bloomsbury Publishing Inc, 1359 Broadway, New York, NY 10018, USA
Bloomsbury Publishing Plc, 50 Bedford Square, London, WC1B 3DP, UK
Bloomsbury Publishing Ireland, 29 Earlsfort Terrace, Dublin 2, D02 AY28, Ireland

First published in the United States of America 2026

Library of Congress Cataloging-in-Publication Data Available

ISBN: HB: 979-8-216-27774-3
ePDF: 979-8-216-27776-7
eBook: 979-8-216-27775-0

Series: Revolutionary Bioethics

Typeset by Integra Software Services Pvt. Ltd.

For product safety-related questions contact productsafety@bloomsbury.com.

To find out more about our authors and books visit www.bloomsbury.com and sign up for our newsletters.

Contents

Tables

Acknowledgments

My special thanks go to Ignacio Mastroleo, Florencia Luna, Erik Malmqvist, and Stéphane Chauvier for their support.

I also thank Patrick Müller.

Part One

Setting the Stage

1

International Health Research and Poor Communities: An Introduction

The Moral Issue at Stake

For decades, research ethics has addressed the standards governing research conducted in low- and middle-income countries (LMICs). Given these countries' economic instability, fragile health and welfare systems, widespread poverty, and regulatory uncertainty, concerns about violations of established ethical norms in research remain particularly pressing (Schroeder et al. 2018).

Research conducted in low-income settings often raises questions about the balance between the benefits accruing to foreign researchers and sponsoring institutions and the benefits reaching host communities in LMICs (Homedes and Ugalde 2015). There are certainly some important benefits for LMIC communities when international health research is conducted in these settings.

First, there is evidence that governments and patients in LMICs welcome sponsors from abroad. This can be explained by the fact that many citizens of LMICs are willing to participate in international health research trials in the hope of receiving treatments that are often unavailable due to poverty and inadequate health care provision (Zvonareva et al. 2015). Governments also hope to attract industry investment and improve infrastructure and employment opportunities, while domestic researchers seek training, increased income, and opportunities to advance local academic systems (Marshall 2008; Normile 2008).

However, the benefits to host communities must be considered in the context of the overall benefits generated. There is a repeated concern that communities benefit disproportionately little. This becomes especially visible when considering the global pharmaceutical market and the structural incentives that shape global health research. It is estimated that the global pharmaceutical market will be worth USD 1.65 trillion in 2024, with projections reaching USD 2.35 trillion by 2030 (Grand View Horizon 2025). In 2024, the North American market accounted for 53 percent of global pharmaceutical sales (EFPIA 2024, 4). Major players such as Pfizer, Novartis, and Roche continue to dominate the market, generating substantial revenues while investing proportionately less in research and development. Consequently, revenues remain concentrated in the pharmaceutical industry in high-income regions (Expert Market Research 2023).

The COVID-19 pandemic illustrated this dynamic quite well. Despite limited funding and infrastructure, LMICs contributed significantly to research on the pandemic and adapted treatments to meet local needs (Holzer et al. 2023a). South Africa, for example, emerged as a leader in vaccine trials, contributing to pivotal research on the AstraZeneca and Johnson & Johnson vaccines. Bangladesh made significant strides in developing affordable, rapid diagnostic kits. Yet the pandemic simultaneously exacerbated existing structural inequalities in global health: LMICs received disproportionately few resources, medical technologies, and vaccine doses relative to high-income countries (Dal-Re et al. 2021; Figueroa et al. 2021; Holzer et al. 2023).

***

Historically, the internationalization of pharmaceutical trials accelerated when LMICs still lacked the safeguards, harmonized research standards, and infrastructure that the industry required. Although trials took place in LMICs during the 1970s and 1980s, the early 1990s marked an era in which the US Food and Drug Administration (FDA)[1] began to actively promote clinical trials in LMICs. The FDA declared that identifying research sites and sources of data abroad would become part of its mandate to determine the safety and efficacy of new medical interventions. The subsequent approval of the *Good*

Clinical Practice (GCP)[2] guidelines in 1996, emerging from an international conference, together with the Agreement on Trade-Related Aspects of Intellectual Property Rights (WTO 2017),[3] provided important regulatory frameworks facilitating the global expansion of clinical research.

Research ethicists Homedes and Ugalde (2014) have shown that, ever since, pharmaceutical companies have increasingly relocated trials to other countries to reduce costs and recruit research participants. Supporting data show that research and development costs can be drastically reduced in LMICs, with costs per patient being 40–90 percent lower than in industrialized countries (Glickman et al. 2009; Homedes and Ugalde 2014, 58). In terms of participant recruitment, the pharmaceutical industry began to require larger populations of test subjects and needed to reduce the time from research to production (Homedes and Ugalde 2014, 57).

To date, a considerable proportion of the pharmaceutical industry's revenue stems from research and drug testing conducted in the Global South. But the resulting distribution of benefits remains deeply unequal: monetary, non-material, and health benefits generated in LMICs predominantly accrue to investigators, sponsors, and countries abroad, rather than to host communities themselves (Homedes and Ugalde 2014; Luna and Holzer 2025; Wenner 2018a).

This unequal distribution is reinforced by the structure of the global pharmaceutical system. Under the international TRIPS agreement, approved drugs are often sold at high prices. Combined with the limited funding available to many LMIC health systems, essential medications remain out of reach for much of the population. As a consequence, roughly half of the world's population is pushed into extreme poverty and lacks access to basic health services (World Bank 2025). Furthermore, research and development efforts continue to focus predominantly on conditions prevalent in high-income countries, where health care markets are most profitable (Chapman et al. 2021; Hollis 2007; Hotez et al. 2022; Pogge 2008, 2009). Diseases that disproportionately affect LMIC populations, including tuberculosis and neglected tropical diseases,[4] remain comparatively underfunded and understudied, leaving critical health needs unmet (Buchanan et al. 2011, 307).

Global Health Research in Low-Income Communities: Setting the Stage

Research as a Collective Enterprise Involving "Host Communities"

Health research, and clinical research in particular, can be understood as a multilateral enterprise in which diverse agents and institutions cooperate in the pursuit of knowledge. At its core, it is an epistemic practice aimed at producing generalizable knowledge of the effects and efficacy of medical interventions (Kimmelman and London 2015, 29–30). Yet, research is never merely a technical procedure. It is a social practice that connects economic interests, institutional authority and oversight, and those involved as researchers, sponsors, and research subjects. In the conduct of a clinical trial, sponsors are the legal entities responsible for initiating, managing, and financing the research. They can be public or private, but in practice are most often pharmaceutical corporations.

The growth of the global pharmaceutical industry has led to the emergence of specialized research intermediaries, so-called Contract Research Organizations (CROs). These legal entities represent a new stage in the internationalization of research. They operate transnationally, coordinating trials for pharmaceutical, biotechnological, or medical device companies that outsource their research processes (Petryna 2009, 24). By 2010, roughly one-third of global research and development funding was administered by CROs (Homedes and Ugalde 2014, 75).

Next to these private actors stand local regulatory bodies and governmental health authorities. They allocate resources for research, oversee ethical review, and regulate national standards of research governance (CIOMS-WHO 2016, commentary on guideline 23). Research ethics committees (RECs) play a central role in this process. Their task is not only to evaluate the scientific standards of research involving human participants but also to safeguard ethical standards (Gelling 1999; Wendler 2017).

The institutionalization of RECs varies considerably across contexts. In many LMICs, systems of ethical review exist formally but lack adequate accreditation, training, or institutional independence. As Homedes and Ugalde (2014) show for Latin America, few countries possess effective systems for evaluating the performance of ethics committees, and regulations often fail to specify essential requirements such as independence from administrative bodies and inclusion of community representatives. Consequently, the environment within which research is conducted is not always characterized by transparency, self-assessment, or systematic oversight.

Research, moreover, always takes place in communities. As defined above, the "host community" is the local population that provides the research site and from which research participants are often recruited. Within this population, a distinction can be drawn between research participants and non-participating community members. Participants directly enroll in studies and thus bear the risks and have possible benefits of experimental interventions. They may, for example, receive access to treatments that are otherwise unavailable, ancillary health care, or post-trial benefits (Richardson 2012). Researchers and sponsors have to comply with strict ethical requirements when recruiting research subjects. For instance, they must ensure voluntary and informed consent, fair subject recruitment, and a reasonable harm-benefit profile, so as to justify the exposure of subjects to potential risks (see Nuremberg Code 1949).

Most scholarship in research ethics has focused on research participants. Yet, as I argue throughout this work, the moral significance of host communities extends beyond those who actively participate in research. While the ethics of research participants has been extensively debated, the moral status of non-participating members of host communities remains comparatively underexplored. Nevertheless, the late 1980s and 1990s saw the emergence of important discussions on this topic (Angell 1988; Angell 1997; Annas and Grodin 1998; Glantz et al. 1998; Goodin 1987; Macklin 2004; Resnik 1998; Varmus and Satcher 1997). These debates began to articulate a view of host communities as moral stakeholders rather than passive bystanders, a position echoed in later ethics frameworks (Emanuel and Participants 2008; Glantz et al. 1998; Participants in the 2001 Conference on Ethical Aspects of Research in Developing Countries 2004). This work will begin from this insight, aiming to explore the moral obligations arising from the recognition of research as a practice embedded within, and dependent upon, host communities.

To proceed, the concept and scope of community itself must be clarified. The literature and existing ethics guidelines reveal two main conceptualizations. The narrow conception understands community as a group of people sharing a locality or characteristic, such as geographical, cultural, or social ties (London 2008; Participants in the 2001 Conference on Ethical Aspects of Research in Developing Countries 2004). Much of the discussion about "local community engagement" appeals to this narrow understanding of community (London 2008).

However, there is a second common understanding of community that I will mainly refer to, which I will call the "broad" conception. The broad conception conceives of communities as groups that share certain attitudes and interests (Oxford Dictionary 2024). This conception captures the intentional attributes of groups. I will argue in Section "International Ethics Frameworks and Guidelines Regulating the Fair Treatment of Host Communities" that most academic work and ethics guidelines addressing the fair treatment of host communities appeal to this broad notion, claiming that research constitutes a collective enterprise in which relevant stakeholders have certain collective interests.

Yet, as the global distribution of benefits and burdens shows, these relationships are far from equal. The gains of global health research tend to accrue disproportionately to high-income countries and the corporations based within them, even when trials are conducted in the Global South. The ethical challenge, therefore, is to articulate a framework that acknowledges the moral standing of host communities as legitimate stakeholders in the production of global health knowledge.

International Ethics Frameworks and Guidelines Regulating the Fair Treatment of Host Communities

International research ethics frameworks and guidelines are designed to guide and regulate the conduct of research. The first such framework, the Nuremberg Code (1949), emerged in direct response to atrocities committed during Nazi medical experiments.[5] It articulated a set of principles intended to prevent ethically indefensible research. These early standards focused predominantly on the rights of research participants, grounding ethical legitimacy in informed consent and the requirement that experiments generate knowledge necessary for the good of society and unobtainable by other means (Nuremberg Code, paragraph 2).

Over the twentieth century, additional frameworks were developed, including the Belmont Report (National Commission 1979),[6] the Declaration of Helsinki (World Medical Association 2013),[7] and the CIOMS Guidelines (Council for International Organizations of Medical Sciences 2016), jointly established by WHO and UNESCO.[8] Together, these documents constitute an evolving corpus of international research ethics. In contemporary legal literature, ethics guidelines are often regarded as customary international law, and many countries have incorporated parts of these guidelines into national legislation (Andanda 2013, 33).

Considering the treatment of host communities, two crucial claims can be extrapolated from these guidelines. First, communities should be understood as groups united by shared interests or values, in line with the broad conception of community. Second, the fair treatment of communities is best interpreted through the principle of equitable benefit-sharing, that is, the just distribution of benefits and burdens arising from research.

***

Fair Benefit-Sharing

The notion of fair benefit-sharing has become a central concept in contemporary research ethics. It expresses the idea that those who contribute to a joint enterprise—whether through participation, provision of resources, or enabling conditions—are entitled to a just share of resulting benefits. In this sense, fair benefit-sharing represents an ethical translation of reciprocity and justice in exchange. Schroeder defines the principle in the context of resource-sharing as "giving a portion of advantages or profits derived from the use of … resources to the resource providers in order to achieve justice in exchange, with particular emphasis on providing benefits to those who may lack reasonable access to the resulting products and services" (Schroeder 2007, 206).

Benefit-sharing does not necessarily imply monetary remuneration. Most frameworks emphasize non-financial forms of benefit: improved health care infrastructure, capacity building, training for local researchers, access to proven interventions, or the strengthening of local institutions (Hurst 2017, 2). The Declaration of Helsinki (WMA 2013, paragraph 20) specifies that benefits may include special assistance to participants or groups involved in research, support for local health services, and the dissemination of scientific and technological knowledge (Hurst 2017, 3; Hurst 2020). Similarly, the International Bioethics Committee (IBC 2015, paragraph 7)[9] defines a benefit as "something that promotes or enhances the well-being of people, both in the material and spiritual sense," encompassing a range of values from financial gain to the promotion of individual and communal good.

In its beginnings, the idea of benefit-sharing entered the international arena with the Convention on Biological Diversity (CBD 1992), introducing the principle of equitable sharing of benefits from the use of genetic resources (CBD 1992; Post 2003; Schroeder 2007). Although originally focused on nonhuman resources, the CBD set a precedent for recognizing the ethical dimension of global resource exchange. Subsequent documents extended this logic to health research. UNESCO's Universal Declaration on Bioethics and Human Rights (2005) emphasized equitable access to medical, scientific, and technological progress, especially for developing countries (UNESCO 2005, 2f). The Declaration of Helsinki (WMA 2013), the IBC report (2015), and the CIOMS-WHO guidelines (2016) incorporated benefit-sharing as a mechanism for preventing exploitation and ensuring a more just distribution of research outcomes (Hurst 2017, 2; Hurst 2020).

Nonetheless, major practical questions remain unresolved. One persistent concern is the identification of responsible agents. While the CIOMS-WHO guidelines (2016, guideline 2) refer generally to "sponsors, researchers, and relevant public health authorities," they do not specify how responsibilities should be allocated or enforced (Zvonareva et al. 2015). Thus, while the normative demand for fairness is clear, mechanisms of accountability remain ambiguous.

***

Host Communities

Interpreting international ethics frameworks reveals that these documents often employ a broad understanding of "host community." Communities are not merely spatially bounded groups but collectives sharing common interests and attitudes. At the upper level of inclusivity, UNESCO's UDBHR (2005) articulates a distributive vision of justice framing benefit-sharing as a human right. Article 15 declares that "benefits resulting from any scientific research and its applications should be shared with society as a whole and within the international community, in particular with developing countries" (UNESCO 2005, Article 15). Here, community is conceived as global in scope. This universalist view, however, faces familiar challenges. Critics argue that defining benefit-sharing as a human right may be too expansive, especially in contexts where more fundamental needs—such as nutrition, sanitation, or basic health care—remain unmet (Hurst 2017; Schroeder 2014, 221).

Other international guidelines address the term "community" differently, often in a more localized sense. For instance, the WMA (2013) states in the Declaration of Helsinki that a "group participating in research" should benefit from it. More specifically, research should address the health needs and priorities of such a "group" with the aim of making benefits available to it (WMA 2013, paragraph 20). Although an inclusion criterion for group members is still missing, it implies that the community is the immediate population of research participants.

The CIOMS-WHO guidelines (2016) offer a broader perspective. Guideline 2 lists potential beneficiaries as "physicians, researchers, policy makers, public health officials, patients, pharmaceutical companies, communities, and/or the populations where research is conducted." Although not clarified further, reference to both communities and populations suggests different scopes: "communities" denote more localized groups, and "populations" refer to the broader social and political context.[10] The guideline's emphasis on "public health," "welfare," and the use of "infrastructure and public resources" indicates that research is embedded within a larger social structure.

There is no single, unequivocal conceptualization of "community" in international research ethics. The term may refer to a small local group, a domestic population, or, in UNESCO's vision, humanity as a whole. Host communities can thus be interpreted at multiple scales: local, national, or global. These varying interpretations have significant implications. Ethical debates surrounding fair benefit-sharing often oscillate between levels: some emphasize local justice, while others link research to broader distributive responsibilities between the Global North and South.

Unresolved normative questions persist: On what grounds should particular groups be considered legitimate stakeholders? Why, and to what extent, do corporations, sponsors, or other agents owe them a share of benefits? An adequate account of fair benefit-sharing must rest upon a normative foundation specifying who counts as a community, what makes them moral stakeholders, and why fairness requires redistribution of benefits. In practice, the most common usage of "host community" aligns with the level of the host country. This pragmatic understanding reflects both research governance and the realities of global health research. Nevertheless, as I argue in the following chapters, a purely national conception remains insufficient. A philosophically adequate account must address the moral relationships that "bind" local, national, or global communities within a shared research enterprise.

Global Health Trials: Cases from History and Modern Challenges

The ethics of clinical trials in LMICs have been widely discussed, especially in response to research considered unethical toward local communities, as seen in several cases from the 1990s. While a detailed history of the ethical ideas debated in academia will be explored in the next chapter, Section "Two Historical Case Studies" focuses on two key cases where communities were at the center of ethical concerns. These cases are important not only because they helped spark the academic discussion on global justice in health research but also because they shaped how scholars thought about ethical standards in international research. Section "Examples of Current Clinical Research and Sponsorship in LMICs" will then look at how these historical cases relate to the current situation of international clinical trials in LMICs today.

Two Historical Case Studies

The global research programs supported by the CDC and NIH in the United States led research ethicists to carefully consider when international research trials could be considered ethical, especially regarding the responsibilities researchers had to ensure host communities receive fair benefits. While numerous trials could be examined, two cases have emerged as central reference points in the literature. Therefore, I consider it useful to outline them at this stage, given that they have shaped ethical debates for decades (Hawkins and Emanuel 2008). The cases have contributed significantly to discussions concerning the distribution of benefits and the prevention of exploitation in global health research. The aim here is to provide the reader with an intuitive understanding of the ethical tensions, particularly the fine line between enabling host communities to benefit and exposing them to potential exploitation. The first case is Hawkins and Emanuel's (2008) account of a hepatitis A vaccine trial in Thailand, the so-called "Havrix trial," followed by an examination of multiple maternal HIV transmission studies in Africa in the 1990s.

The Havrix Trial

The Havrix inactivated hepatitis A vaccine was tested in 1990 on schoolchildren in Kamphaeng Phet province, Northern Thailand, in a collaborative study sponsored by the Walter Reed Army Institute of Research (US Department of Defense), SmithKline Beecham Biologicals, and Thailand's Ministry of Public Health.[11] The trial began as a Phase 2[12] randomized, double-blind clinical trial involving 300 children, primarily relatives of health care workers, to assess safety and immunogenicity. Following positive results, a larger Phase 3 trial involving 40,000 children aged one to sixteen was conducted with a hepatitis B vaccine control. The study received approval from local and national authorities, including ethics committees and institutional review boards.

Hawkins and Emanuel (2008) explain that the trial was conducted in Thailand due to the high hepatitis A transmission rate (119 per 100,000 population) and previous research infrastructure from a Japanese encephalitis vaccine study. However, there was no formal agreement to make Havrix widely available in Thailand. Budget constraints and prioritization of other vaccines, such as hepatitis B, meant hepatitis A immunization was unlikely to be included in national programs. The US government and SmithKline Beecham Biologicals did not commit to providing Havrix at no cost, though the company verbally agreed to pursue vaccine registration for private market sales, targeting travelers from developed countries rather than the Thai population.

Despite limited access to Havrix, the trial offered other benefits. Participants received hepatitis B vaccines and potentially the hepatitis A vaccine. Additionally, medical services were improved, health workers were trained, and public health stations were upgraded with refrigeration, medicines, and supplies. Schools hosting the trial received improved sanitary facilities, and 2,500 teachers, health workers, and officials involved in the study were vaccinated against hepatitis B. Training for Thai researchers aimed to enhance clinical trial expertise for future vaccine studies, including an HIV vaccine trial.

However, the study faced criticism from Thai scientists and the media. Critics argued the trial did not address Thailand's pressing health needs, serving instead the interests of the US Army and affluent travelers. They also highlighted inadequate technology transfer and capacity-building for Thai researchers and the absence of commitments to provide Havrix at reduced costs. These concerns led to allegations that Thai children were exploited for the benefit of wealthier nations. According to an interview with one of the researchers (Hawkins and Emanuel 2008, 58, Interview with Professor Natth 1999), the government ministers agreed with this in private, "... but the sway of international politics and money was too persuasive."

African HIV Maternal Transmission Trials: "The 076 Regimen"

The 076 regimen, introduced in 1994, was the first major breakthrough in reducing maternal-fetal HIV transmission.[13] Developed through the AIDS Clinical Trial Group (ACTG) Study 076, it involved a complex and expensive use of AZT (zidovudine), administered over a strict schedule. Pregnant HIV-infected women began taking oral AZT five times daily during the second trimester for at least twelve weeks. During labor, they received AZT intravenously, and their newborns were given oral AZT four times daily for six weeks. This intensive regimen reduced HIV transmission rates from 25 percent to 8 percent, a groundbreaking 70 percent reduction. However, its cost—averaging $1,000 per woman—made it prohibitive in many parts of the world, particularly in developing countries where annual health care budgets per person were far lower.

In the United States, the discovery was swiftly adopted as the standard of care for HIV-positive pregnant women. However, most HIV-infected women lived—and continue to live—in developing nations with far fewer resources. In countries like Uganda, annual health care spending in the mid-1990s was less than $3 per person. The cost of the 076 regimen was out of reach, and other barriers further complicated implementation. Many women in these regions did not seek prenatal care until late in their pregnancies, if at all, making it difficult to administer the full 076 protocol. Additionally, most women relied on breastfeeding because they could not afford baby formula or lacked access to clean water to prepare it. Breastfeeding, however, was strictly forbidden under the 076 regimen due to the risk of HIV transmission.

Recognizing the urgent need for an affordable and feasible alternative, the World Health Organization (WHO) launched sixteen randomized controlled trials (RCTs) across developing nations, including Uganda, Kenya, Tanzania, and Thailand. These trials tested shorter, simpler AZT regimens to determine if they could effectively reduce transmission while being more practical for resource-limited settings. Fifteen of the trials used placebo controls, sparking ethical controversy. Critics argued that these trials violated the principle of "clinical equipoise," which requires uncertainty about whether a treatment is better than the alternative. Since the effectiveness of AZT had already been proven, withholding it from the control groups was seen as unethical. Furthermore, the trials denied participants access to the best available standard of care provided in sponsoring countries like the United States.

Proponents of the trials, including the Centers for Disease Control and Prevention (CDC), defended the use of placebo controls as necessary for scientific rigor. They argued that historical comparisons were unreliable because many women had not received prenatal care previously, and comparing simplified regimens to the expensive 076 regimen would have required larger trials and longer evaluation times. The CDC and WHO maintained that the trials were designed to address a critical research question: whether affordable regimens could achieve similar efficacy in preventing HIV transmission. Initial findings suggested that the simplified regimens could reduce costs to around $50 per woman. However, this was still unaffordable for many developing nations, where health care spending per person was often far below that figure.

However, Glantz et al. (1998, 3–4) put forward an important critique against the HIV transmission studies. In his view, the ethical acceptability of the studies would have depended on whether the research hypothesis potentially could have yielded benefits for a host country after the trial was finished. Accordingly, the research question should have been formulated as follows:

1. We know that a given regimen of AZT will reduce the rate of maternal-child transmission of HIV.
2. Maternal-child transmission of HIV in many African countries is a serious problem, but the effective AZT regimen is not available because it is too expensive.
3. If an effective AZT regimen costs $X, then it will be made available in the country in which it is to be studied.
4. Therefore, we will conduct trials in certain African countries to see if $X worth of AZT will effectively reduce maternal-to-child transmission of HIV in those countries. (Glantz et al. 1998, 3)

According to Glantz et al. (1998), researchers and sponsors would have necessarily needed to focus on research question (3), as without knowing what dollar amount X actually represented, it was impossible to determine whether the tested intervention would have led to an effective implementation strategy of the intervention and its benefits for the host communities. According to the CDC (1997), the new regimen could have been made available at $50 instead of the previous $800 to $1000 under the 076 regimen.

In this regard, it seemed futile to provide an effective treatment to communities where the annual health expenses per person remained under $10. In Glantz's words:

> If a study found, for example, that \$50 worth of AZT has the same effect as \$800 worth of AZT, it would greatly benefit the *developed world*. Developed countries, which currently spend \$800 per case on drugs alone, could pay substantially less for this preventive measure, and, because the research was conducted elsewhere, none of their citizens would have been put at any risk. At the same time, if the *underdeveloped country* could not afford to spend \$50 any more than it could spend \$800, then it could not possibly derive information that would be of any benefit to its population. (Glantz et al. 1998, 4, emphasis added)

Examples of Current Clinical Research and Sponsorship in LMICs

The landscape of health research in LMICs has changed in the past decade. While the early debates on global research started from the premise that HICs used LMICs solely as recruitment sites to test "drugs on the global poor," some LMICs have now become increasingly sophisticated research ecosystems. Local academic institutions, together with domestic pharmaceutical companies and public-private partnerships, have begun to work together with multinational corporations and foreign sponsors. Domestic research in LMICs is a new phenomenon that has considerably changed the research landscape, especially in middle-income countries like China and India. However, as the following examples will demonstrate, the fundamental issue remains the unequal distribution of funding, benefits and access to resulting innovations for many LMIC communities.

The Persistence of HIC-Sponsored Trials

A significant portion of clinical research in LMICs continues to be led and financed by organizations based in the United States and Western Europe. These studies are often large, late-phase trials seeking to demonstrate efficacy and safety in populations with high disease burden. Regarding the sharing of benefits and access to drugs, recent examples also show that local communities, where drugs are tested, remain systematically excluded from yielding the fruits of research.

Consider, for example, the development of dengue vaccines. Dengue is a mosquito-borne infectious disease across the Global South, especially in South Asia and South America (WHO 2024). The global incidence of dengue has surged dramatically, with over six million cases reported in 2023 and nearly five million by mid-2024 alone (European Centre for Disease Prevention and Control 2024; George et al. 2024). Traditionally, dengue was confined to the Global South, but recent years have seen a rise in autochthonous cases in developed countries. In 2023, 122 cases were reported in Europe, doubling the number seen in 2022 (Brem et al. 2024). Climate change plays a significant role in the spread of vector-borne diseases, as temperature impacts both the life cycle and survival of mosquitoes (Rocklöv and Tozan 2019).

The French pharmaceutical company Sanofi developed *Dengvaxia*, a vaccine designed to prevent severe dengue in individuals who have previously been infected (seropositive). Clinical trials conducted in Latin America and South Asia demonstrated the vaccine's effectiveness in reducing severe disease. However, despite these trials being carried out in the Global South, *Dengvaxia* is primarily available in the United States and Europe, with limited access in Latin American and South Asian countries, where dengue remains a major public health challenge (Tully and Griffiths 2021).

At the close of 2023, the World Health Organization's Strategic Advisory Group of Experts on Immunization (SAGE) approved *Qdenga*, a vaccine created by the Japanese pharmaceutical company Takeda, for the primary prevention of dengue, including among individuals at risk of initial infection, in areas with high dengue transmission and burden. Currently, it is available only in Indonesia, Brazil, and Europe, even though clinical trials were also conducted in other Latin American and South Asian countries (Alves 2024; WHO 2024).

The dengue vaccine case highlights how climate change-related diseases garner research interest from the Global North, with LMICs frequently serving as primary study populations, also nowadays. Funding often favors marketable products such as vaccines, driven by the economic interests of large pharmaceutical companies, which can result in limited accessibility of these interventions in the most affected regions (Global Forum on Bioethics in Research 2024).

However, there might to be other examples that, at first glance, address global disease burden for many people living in LMICs better. To address the ongoing HIV burden, *Gilead Sciences* conducted clinical trials to test the long-acting injectable *Lenacapavir* for HIV pre-exposure prophylaxis. Thousands of women and girls enrolled in sub-Saharan Africa, including sites in Uganda and South Africa, and Latin America, including sites in Argentina, Brazil, Mexico, and Peru, as well as the United States. These Phase 3 trials were unblinded early after demonstrating strong efficacy, and the results have since influenced global policy and WHO guidance on HIV prevention, earning *Lenacapavir* the reputation of a "miraculous drug" (Schütz 2025; Giled 2024). However, while these studies show that large, well-resourced trials can take place successfully in LMICs, they still highlight a structural imbalance: Despite the efforts by Gilead Sciences to make lenacapivir available through tiered pricing policies and a nonexclusive voluntary licensing agreement and technology transfer to six generic manufacturers—a major step toward making the drug accessible—the Access to Medicines Foundation (2025) highlights major outstanding concerns: particularly the lack of access for seventeen LMICs excluded from the license, which together accounted for nearly one-fifth of new HIV infections in 2023 (Access to Medicines Foundation 2025).

These examples illustrate that, although there is growing pressure on the global pharmaceutical industry to share benefits, and some initiatives demonstrate genuine intent to improve access, it remains uncertain whether local communities actually receive a fair share of the benefits from drug testing—particularly the poorest populations.

Domestically Sponsored Trials in LMICs

Compared to the 1990s, some LMICs have undergone a significant transformation and successfully established research infrastructures and emerged as major domestic sponsors of clinical trials. China and India provide prominent examples of this shift.

Since regulatory reforms in the late 2010s, China's domestic companies have dominated the country's clinical trial landscape. Industry analysts estimate that 85–95 percent of new drug trials in China are sponsored by Chinese firms rather than multinationals (Hankun Law 2023; Hart 2024). This shift has ultimately been driven by state investment in biotech, the emergence of national contract research organizations, and streamlined regulatory pathways. A recent example is the approval granted to CSPC Pharmaceutical Group in mid-2024 to initiate human trials of its novel mRNA cancer therapy, SYS6020 (Silver 2024).

Regarding India, the rapid mobilization of its manufacturing industry in the pharmaceutical sector was demonstrated during the COVID-19 pandemic. The vaccines Bharat Biotech's *Covaxin* and Zydus Cadila's *ZyCoV-D* were developed and tested in India, with support from domestic research institutions and the Indian Council of Medical Research. These programs progressed through all three clinical phases domestically, with data submitted to Indian regulators and published in peer-reviewed journals (Bharat Biotech 2021; Zydus Cadila 2021). While Covaxin was later authorized in ninety-six countries, ZyCoV-D remained a domestically used product (Business Standard 2021; Livemint 2021). Beyond vaccines, Indian sponsors have expanded into areas such as oncology and metabolic disorders (Shinde et al. 2023). This domestic sponsorship supports local capacity building, regulatory expertise, and regionally relevant innovation. Yet, funding and infrastructure disparities between urban research hubs and rural regions remain substantial (Basu 2022).

South–South and LMIC Partnerships

More recently, South-South partnerships have emerged beyond national boundaries, involving NGO and academic leadership in their establishment. South-South partnerships refer to cooperative arrangements among LMICs to advance shared development goals and also to exchange knowledge, technology, and resources.

For instance, collaborative consortia in Africa have tested interventions for malaria, maternal health, and antimicrobial resistance through shared governance structures (Marcad Consortium n.d.; Tagoe et al. 2023). Brazil and China have collaborated on vaccine production and technology transfer during the pandemic, with the Instituto Butantan testing the Chinese Sinovac vaccine in a Phase 3 study in Brazil (Instituto Butantan 2021). India and South

Africa have established long-standing pharmaceutical partnerships to expand generic antiretroviral production ('t Hoen 2018). There are also regional initiatvies in place: the African Union's Partnership for African Vaccine Manufacturing and ASEAN public-health cooperation further demonstrate how South-South collaboration can strengthen local manufacturing, improve outbreak response, and enhance health system resilience (African Union 2021; Caballero-Anthony 2018).

The Chinese vaccine producers Sinovac and Sinopharm sponsored multicountry COVID-19 vaccine studies in several countries, most of them LMICs in Asia, Africa, and Latin America (New Drug Approvals 2021; Sinovac Press Release 2021). This outward expansion marks a reversal of the traditional flow of research sponsorship: LMIC firms are increasingly exporting technology and conducting pivotal trials in other LMIC markets.

Aim and Road Ahead

Developing a Normative Model

The central aim of this book is to develop and defend a normative account of how global health research ought to address the interests of communities in low-income settings. Building on the introductory remarks and the case examples, I focus on two interrelated questions:

i. Why do researchers and sponsors bear obligations toward host communities? (Justification requirement)
ii. If such obligations exist, what is their content? (Content requirement)

Any ethical account that fails to address both questions is incomplete. A normative framework must provide both a robust moral justification for obligations and clear guidance regarding the content of those obligations. The justification requirement concerns the moral grounds for treating host communities as legitimate stakeholders in research. This entails a clear conceptualization of community membership and the identification of individuals and groups that hold claims to the fruits of research. While much of the literature assumes the legitimacy of host communities as stakeholders, I contend that this assumption is not self-evident and requires rigorous conceptual justification.

The content requirement addresses the normative question of what constitutes a "fair benefit" and how to determine its proper distribution. The Havrix trial illustrates the complexity of this question. In this case, benefits included the tested hepatitis A vaccine, hepatitis B immunization, capacity building, and modernization of local infrastructure. Opinions about the content of benefits diverged. Some considered forms of capacity building to be fair benefits, while others criticized the exclusion of the host population from therapeutic benefits of the tested drug. This case highlights a critical normative issue: Should fair benefits be limited to outcomes directly related to the intervention under study, or may they include broader contributions such as infrastructure, education, or financial support? A normative account must clarify these distinctions and provide principled guidance for resolving them.

In the following chapters, I will develop an account that aligns with what Maria Merritt (2011) frames as a normative model in research ethics: a "systemic, critically reflective, and practically useful account of a moral obligation" (2011, 313). A successful normative model in research ethics should be able to frame and guide deliberation by offering the following three things:

> (1) It should provide a principled basis for determining whether, for what reasons, and under what conditions researchers [and sponsors] have any … obligation; (2) it should non-arbitrarily specify the content of any such obligation, that is, what kinds of … needs (if any) researchers [and sponsors] have an obligation to address; and (3) it should non-arbitrarily locate lower and upper limits on the extent of any such obligation. (Merritt 2011, 314)

Applied to global health research and the fair treatment of communities, a normative model should provide both justification for obligations to host communities and guidance regarding the content of those obligations, derived from an underlying set of normative principles. Crucially, the model should indicate what counts as the discharge of an obligation, including minimal and potentially maximal requirements.

Obligations in my framework will be conceptualized as special and perfect. Special obligations are "owed to some subset of persons," in contrast to natural duties that are "owed to all persons simply qua persons" (Jeske 2021). Common-sense morality understands us as having special obligations to those with whom we stand in some sort of special relationship or those to whom we have made promises or commitments of some sort (Jeske 2021). I here particularly assume that special obligations arise from interactions among different parties, maintaining that the nature of the interaction puts individuals in different special relationships. This stands in contrast to universal duties as moral requirements which are owed by "all persons to all others" (Sidgwick 1907, 13; Simmons 1979a, b).

Obligations can be characterized not only as special but also as perfect requirements. Perfect duties admit "of no exception in favor of inclination" to refrain from acting on a maxim. Imperfect duties, by contrast, require us to pursue acts that can admit of exceptions and are thus owed to no one in particular (Johnson and Cureton 2016; O'Neill 1996).

The Main Argument in Brief and Chapter Overview

In line with the central aim of this book, I will briefly outline the core argument. The first substantive part, *Transactions*, critically examines existing normative accounts—which I will summarize as *transactional normative models*—and demonstrates why they inadequately address both the justification and content requirements for fair benefit-sharing. These normative models, advanced by prominent authors such as Ezekiel Emanuel (2008), the participants of the 2001 Conference on Ethical Aspects of Research in Developing Countries (Emanuel and Participants 2008; Participant 2004), Rebecca Wolitz et al. (2009), Ruth Macklin (2004, 2011), Alex John London (2008), Bridget Pratt, Adnan A. Hyder (2014), and other contemporary authors, remain influential in research ethics literature. My critique focuses on their insufficient development of the *justification argument*, particularly their failure to provide a normative foundation for community-wide fairness obligations. A central problem lies in their lack of conceptual clarity regarding host communities and in establishing these communities as legitimate moral stakeholders.

The second substantive part, *Fair Play*, proposes an alternative normative framework that engages with existing ethics guidelines and the broader debates surrounding community engagement, fair benefit-sharing, and exploitation in global research. Importantly, this model does not seek to overturn the moral history or practice of global research ethics but instead aims to address the shortcomings of current approaches while providing a normative foundation for both the *justification* and *content* of fair benefit-sharing.

The *fair play model* conceptualizes research as a cooperative enterprise oriented toward producing socially valuable epistemic outputs, i.e., knowledge capable of curing, alleviating, or preventing disease. Within this cooperative framework, host communities are recognized as relevant stakeholders, owing to their contributions to the success of research. This argument draws on Robert A. Phillips' (1997) adaptation of John Rawls' (1964, 1971, 1999a) well-known principle of fairness, or *fair play*, which identifies legitimate claims to benefits among those who restrict their liberty and incur burdens to support the cooperative endeavor. Conversely, beneficiaries of the research are morally obligated to contribute their fair share.

A central contribution of the fair play model is that it addresses both the justification and content requirements of fair benefit-sharing. Additionally, I demonstrate that another set of normative alternatives to transactional models, that is, cosmopolitan models, address general duties (often more demanding) but fail to account for special obligations. My framework thus offers a third alternative that accounts for *special obligations* arising within cooperative schemes.

I shall now offer a brief overview of the chapters to set the stage for what follows. The book proceeds by guiding the reader from the conceptual foundations of the problem, through critical analysis of existing approaches, toward the articulation of the *fair play model.*

Chapter 2 traces the genealogy of key concepts, that is, "fair benefits," "community exploitation," and the "social value requirement." These concepts emerged in response to ethical concerns about double standards between high- and low-income countries, particularly during HIV transmission studies in the 1990s. This chapter critiques the lack of normative justification and proposes a framework for moving forward.

Chapter 3 reconstructs two dominant normative models in research ethics—the *vulnerability model* and the *economic model*—both rooted in a *transactional paradigm*. These models conceptualize fairness obligations through individual transactions but fail on three counts:

i. They inadequately define obligations toward host communities. This further implies that transactional models cannot account for what many authors call "community exploitation."
ii. The ethical models neglect structural injustices beyond individual transactions.
iii. The economic model's reliance on market fairness undermines the achievement of fair benefits (noncompliance with the content requirement).

Chapter 4 introduces the fair play model as an alternative to transactional approaches (objection i). Host communities, as collaborators in producing socially valuable knowledge, acquire moral claims to benefits. Obligations to fairly share benefits arise from the cooperative enterprise, grounded in the "principle of fairness." Exploitation occurs when communities contribute but receive insufficient benefits, allowing researchers and sponsors to free-ride on the cooperative efforts of communities.

Chapter 5 extends the model to include affluent beneficiaries of research, primarily in high-income countries. The fair play model maintains that fairness obligations apply to all agents who derive substantial benefits from the cooperative enterprise, which stays in contrast with cosmopolitan theories that impose general duties rather than context-specific obligations.

Chapter 6 links community exploitation to structural injustices in health research (objection ii). Structural factors enable exploitative practices, such as conducting low-cost trials in settings with double standards. The fair play model emphasizes addressing these background injustices to ensure fair cooperation and prevent exploitation.

Chapter 7 focuses on the content requirement (objection iii), proposing an alternative to transactional models for defining fair benefits. It explores distributive principles like Rawls' *difference principle* and frameworks like *accountability for reasonableness*. The chapter also addresses concrete applications of those principles and their institutional mechanisms to ensure fair benefits, and specifically research taxes, patent reforms, prior agreements, and efforts of improving transparency.

Chapter 8 revisits the cases introduced in Chapter 1 in light of the conceptual and normative framework developed in previous chapters. It further addresses two major objections commonly discussed in research ethics literature: (i) The *non-worseness constraint*, which raises the concern that enforcing fair benefit-sharing could deter research in low-income settings, reducing the overall benefits available to mainly poor populations; (ii) the risk of *undue inducement*, where excessive benefits offered to host communities might coerce participation and compromise autonomy.

Part Two

Transactions

2

From the "Double Standard" to "Fair Benefits," "Community Exploitation," and the "Social Value Requirement"

A Short History of International Health Research Ethics

Despite the wide recognition outside the United States of the Belmont Report launched in 1979 and the US regulatory framework for research with human beings, also known as the "Common Rule," many ethicists, researchers, and health authorities requested a more international perspective. Back then, the Council for International Organizations and Medical Sciences (CIOMS)—founded in 1949 as a joint association between the World Health Organization (WHO) and the United Nations Scientific and Cultural Organization (UNESCO) with the aim of facilitating and promoting international biomedical research—already existed. In the late 1970s, CIOMS in association with WHO undertook its work on the ethics of biomedical research, which resulted in the publication of "Proposed International Ethical Guidelines for Biomedical Research Involving Human Subjects" in 1982. At the time, newly independent WHO member states were setting up health care systems, but the WHO did not promote ethics as an aspect of health care and research. Thus, CIOMS set out, in cooperation with the WHO, to prepare guidelines indicating how general ethical principles should guide biomedical research involving human subjects, particularly in developing countries, where socioeconomic circumstances, laws, and regulations differed from those in high-income countries (HICs). These ethical principles were previously set forth in the World Medical Association's Declaration of Helsinki in 1964 and in an amended version in 1975 (CIOMS-WHO 2002).

Medical researchers from developed countries performed most of their experiments during the 1970s on fellow citizens, frequently choosing subjects from poor and vulnerable subpopulations, including prisoners in the United States (Petryna 2009, 23). With the beginning of the global HIV epidemic in the 1980s, research began to gain international reach. Populations in sub-Saharan Africa were thought to be suitable for large-scale studies where patient populations at risk for HIV infection could be easily identified. The harmonization of technical requirements for the registration of pharmaceuticals for human use as well as a harmonized international patent system under the TRIPS regime in the 1990s facilitated this trend (Petryna 2009, 24–37).

Yet, the National Institutes of Health (NIH) in the United States and the American and European investigators conducting more and more globalized studies were unfamiliar with the culture, customs, and economic pressures in their new research environment (Angell 1988; Barry 1988). Thus, it seemed that large-scale trials in the developing world together with rapid advances in medicine and biotechnology, changing research practices such as multinational field trials, and also the view that research was largely beneficial to "vulnerable" groups, gave rise to new ethical questions and views (CIOMS-WHO 2002). In response, the CIOMS-WHO released the *International Ethical Guidelines for Biomedical Research Involving Human Subjects* in 1993, which was updated in 2002 and 2016 and is one of the most influential publications regulating international health research with human subjects, even up to the present day (see Chapter 1). The CIOMS-WHO guidelines (1993) acknowledged for the first time in the history of research ethics the conduct of externally sponsored clinical trials as a reaction to globalized health research landscapes and specifically addressed the obligations of the sponsoring party and host countries:

Externally sponsored research entails two ethical obligations:

> An external sponsoring agency should submit the research protocol to ethical and scientific review according to the standards of the country of the sponsoring agency, and the ethical standards applied should be no less exacting than they would be in the case of research carried out in that country.

> After scientific and ethical approval in the country of the sponsoring agency, the appropriate authorities of the host country, including a national or local ethical review committee or its equivalent, should satisfy themselves that the proposed research meets their own ethical requirements. (CIOMS-WHO 1993, guideline 15)

By "externally sponsored research," CIOMS-WHO (1993) meant research undertaken in a host country but sponsored, financed, and sometimes wholly or partly carried out by an external sponsor. In a comment on guideline 15, CIOMS-WHO (1993) explicitly stated that committees in sponsoring countries or international agencies had special responsibilities to carry out research that was sound and suitable in terms of safety, provided favorable risk-benefit ratios, and offered a sound "justification for conducting the research in the host country rather than in the country of the sponsoring agency." The conduct of research in the host society should, under no circumstances, violate the current ethical standards of the sponsoring country. Moreover, the host countries were assigned the task of determining whether the goals of the research would be responsive to their health needs and priorities.

In the same vein and probably as a response to the 1993 CIOMS-WHO guidelines, the World Medical Association (WMA) wrote in its 1996 Declaration of Helsinki:

> In any medical study, every patient—including those of a control group, if any—should be assured of the best proven diagnostic and therapeutic method. This does not exclude the use of inert placebo in studies where no proven diagnostic or therapeutic method exists. (WMA 1996, II.3)

The early drafts of both documents show that from the beginning, those thinking critically about international health research in LMIC contexts were clearly in favor of a "no double standard" approach to international trials. The no double standard requirement means that the best proven diagnostic and therapeutic methods ought to be standard for any kind of research enterprise. Ethical standards should not be lower in LMIC trials compared to trials conducted in the developed world where ethical guidelines are more rigorously enforced. External sponsoring agencies were moreover identified as the agents responsible for developing and ensuring host countries' capacities to conduct research without resort to a double standard and for leaving some sort of positive impact on their development and health system (see London 2005). Subsequently, in "Ethical Imperialism?" (1988), Marcia Angell argued against ethical relativism and defended the claim that ethical standards should be seen as universal.

Despite the regulatory frameworks developed in the 1990s, the reality of the past decades suggests that international researchers and sponsors have hardly complied with the strict ethical requirements set by the CIOMS-WHO (1993) guidelines and the Declaration of Helsinki (WMA 1996). The African HIV transmission studies in the 1990s (Glantz et al. 1998; Varmus and Satcher 1997) and the Havrix trial (Hawkins and Emanuel 2008, chap. 2) are only two representative examples in the 1990s of widely and publicly discussed research cases that failed to comply with the no double standard requirement. Here, it should be added that the double standard was not due to any lack of capacity on the part of Western researchers and sponsors to provide active controls. The issue was the perception that rich sponsors and investigators took undue advantage of populations in countries that were affected by socioeconomic injustices (CIOMS-WHO 2002). Thus, the aforementioned trials triggered a new debate about the use of placebo controls and the possibility of accepting a double standard in offshored health research.

Some of the first authors who commented on the HIV transmission studies in Africa were Lurie and Wolfe (1997) from the Public Citizen's Health Research Group and Angell (1997). Macklin (2004, 2008) and London (2008) followed them by pointing to the unethical design of the Surfaxin trial. Lurie and Wolfe wrote a letter to US Secretary of Health and Human Services Donna Shalala and published a commentary in the *New England Journal of Medicine*. Marcia Angell, the executive editor of the journal, published simultaneously an editorial supporting Lurie and Wolfe's position, comparing the African HIV transmission studies to the infamous Tuskegee studies in which African Americans were refused treatment for syphilis (Hawkins and Emanuel 2008). By appealing to the CIOMS-WHO guidelines that prohibited a double standard in research, Lurie and Wolfe (1997) as well as Angell (1997) argued for better ethical standards and against the unethical employment of randomized controlled trials in all cases where effective treatments were available.

At the same time and in stark contrast to these efforts, Harold Varmus of the NIH and David Satcher of the Centers for Disease Control and Prevention (CDC) defended research studies performed under a double standard. They specifically addressed the HIV transmission studies, which were supported by the NIH and the CDC (see Chapter 1). They mounted their defense in a comment on the HIV transmission studies in *The New England Journal of Medicine* (1997), outlining the rationale of the NIH and CDC in sponsoring the trials. The comment suggests that the NIH and CDC both actively tried to support science, participation in the ethics review, and public health in the respective host countries. Regarding the placebo use, they argued that alternative trial designs were carefully considered. In their view, the placebo-controlled studies provided a faster and more definite answer about safety and efficacy with fewer subjects and with less aggressive subject enrollment (Varmus and Satcher 1997, 3005). The authors thus felt that the trials were ethically legitimate, as placebo controls were necessary in order to gain the knowledge sought, and no participant was made worse off by participating in the trial (Hawkins and Emanuel 2008).

In sum, we may say that the debate about the ethics of research trials in low and middle-income contexts started in the mid-1990s when commentators discussed the double standard in research. Two prominent bioethics journals, *Bioethics* and the *Hastings Center Report*, devoted whole issues to the debate, with articles defending both sides (see, e.g., volume 12, issue 4 (1998) of Bioethics and the volume 28, issue 6 (1998) of Hastings Center Report; Hawkins and Emanuel 2008, 17). In the end, it seemed the defenders of a double standard got the edge on their critics. As Hawkins and Emanuel (2008) argue, many significant health policy groups, including UNAIDS, CIOMS, the Nuffield Council, and the US National Bioethics Advisory Commission (NBAC), abandoned the "best proven treatment" condition set in the Declaration of Helsinki (WMA 1996) in the early 2000s.

From the "Double Standard" to "Exploitation" and "the Social Value Requirement"

In their 1997 comment, Varmus and Satcher put forward the intuition that research would need to serve the health needs of *host populations*. This argument turned away from the no double standard requirement, which concerned the benefits to individual research subjects, and instead spotlighted the importance of benefiting host countries and obtaining "in-country participation." Varmus and Satcher held that "trials that make use of impoverished populations to test drugs for use solely in developed countries violate our most basic understanding of ethical behavior" (Varmus and Satcher 1997, 1003).

Despite widespread condemnation of the design of the HIV transmission trials, Varmus and Satcher denied that researchers and the external sponsoring agencies, the NIH and the CDC, would have conducted a study without adequately addressing the host communities' health needs. In the following years, two important concepts—*exploitation* and the *social value requirement*—came to dominate the research ethics literature in response to Varmus and Satcher's viewpoint.

Exploitation

Glantz et al. (1998) replied to Varmus and Satcher's statement by criticizing the HIV transmission trials as an absurd attempt to offer a feasible and sustainable long-term solution for the provision of the tested drug Zidovudine (AZT) in African countries. This critique was no longer related to the no double standard requirement, but another ethical concern, namely, exploitation. According to the authors, research practices that (i) do not address the health needs of a community and/or (ii) do not lead to the implementation of the medical intervention under testing qualify as exploitative. The latter condition was discussed as "reasonable availability" in the CIOMS-WHO guidelines from 1993. Moreover, in order to comply with reasonable availability, interventions would need to be affordable and presuppose an appropriate health infrastructure to deliver the tested drug or intervention to the local people. Thus, Glantz et al. (1998) emphasized the affordability constraint of reasonable availability in addition to the condition that research ought to be relevant to a local population's health needs. Exploitation occurs when communities cannot derive information from a trial that would be of benefit to them and when this information, in turn, primarily benefits developed nations. This is a concern beyond the avoidance of double standards. To make this point explicit, Glantz et al. (1998) highlighted the ethical deficits of the HIV transmission trials, as follows:

> If a study found, for example, that $50 worth of AZT has the same effect as $800 worth of AZT, it would greatly benefit the developed world. Developed countries, which currently spend $800 per case on drugs alone, could pay substantially less for this preventive measure, and, because the research was conducted elsewhere, none of their citizens would have been put at any risk. At the same time, if the underdeveloped country could not afford to spend $50 any more than it could spend $800, then it could not possibly derive information that would be of any benefit to its population. This is the definition of exploitation. (Glantz et al. 1998, 3)

As depicted in Table 2.1, a research trial aiming for the generation of information that is not of use to a developing community—because the drugs

Table 2.1 1990s African HIV Transmission Trials: Reconstruction of an Argument by Glantz et al. (1998), *drawn from Glantz et al. (1998)*

	Interventions	
	AZT long course	AZT short course (under testing)
Cost of the intervention	$800	$50
Affordable for the United States and other developed countries?	Yes	Yes
Affordable for African countries participating in the trials?	No	No. The per capita health care expenditures of most of the African countries involved in mother-to-child HIV transmission prevention trials ranged in the 1990s from $5 to $22 (Glantz et al 1998: note 11)

will be unaffordable regardless of the research outcome—exploits host populations. Testing whether a short course of $50 AZT can be used to inhibit mother-to-child HIV transmission only provides value for those countries and communities that can afford to pay this price. In addition, research is ethically unjustified in the absence of a plan to improve a country's health care delivery capabilities. In many cases, international research trials have been conducted in poor communities that are vulnerable in the sense that they cannot protect themselves against such exploitative practices. External researchers and sponsoring agencies would be therefore required to uphold effective targeting of health needs and to provide an effective implementation strategy for the tested medical intervention prior to beginning a trial (Glantz et al. 1998: 3).

Annas and Grodin (1998) aligned with the general subtext laid out in Glantz et al.'s argumentation. In their view, the central issue at stake in externally sponsored trials in low- and middle-income countries is exploitation. Researchers and sponsors can prevent exploitation when they ensure that an intervention proven to be effective is delivered to a host community. To do this, high-income countries would need to implement programs to promote the health of people in developing countries by improving the public health infrastructure and by delivering effective drugs and vaccines to people (Annas and Grodin 1998, 561–2).

Exploitation and the Social Value Requirement

Almost at the same time, another concept emerged in the discussion. Glantz and colleagues (1998) argued that in order to be justifiable research would need to offer the potential of actual benefit to the inhabitants of developing countries, meaning that host countries should be able to derive sufficient information from a research proposal to judge whether it is appropriate to implement a candidate intervention. A few years later, Emanuel and colleagues published papers entitled "What Makes Clinical Research Ethical?" (2000) and "What Makes Clinical Research in Developing Countries Ethical?" (2004), in which they offered a systematic account of the common consensus that research is ethically permissible only if certain principles are fulfilled. The "social value of knowledge principle," more commonly known as the "social value requirement" (Wendler and Rid 2017; Wenner 2015, 2018a), is one of these guiding principles.

The most recent version of the CIOMS-WHO guidelines (2016) considers the social value requirement to be the fundamental principle underpinning the ethical justification of any biomedical research project involving humans. According to paragraph 1 of the CIOMS-WHO (2016), research is the prospect of generating knowledge in terms of some expected social utility (see Wenner 2015, 2018a) or the means to protect and promote people's health and welfare. The anticipated epistemic results of research justify the performance of the experiment as long as the knowledge produced is not procurable by other methods or means.[1]

Wendler and Rid (2017) deem the social value to be a minimal requirement: clinical research must have *sufficient* social value, which means that research without at least some valuable epistemic output for a host community cannot be ethically justified. However, the social value of research does not mandate that the social value of all clinical trials must exceed some threshold for significance or importance (Wendler and Rid 2017, 78–9). Wenner (2015) complements this view by arguing that, applied to a specific context, the social value requirement offers a general prima facie justification to conduct a research study in a certain host community. She concludes that "what is ethically troubling about some cases is that all of the epistemic value produced accrues to populations who do not share the same social context as those undertaking risk for the sake of its generation" (Wenner 2015, 82).

As pointed out in the last section, if developed countries use inhabitants of a developing country to obtain new significant knowledge and create products that are beneficial to both developing and developed countries, but only developed countries gain access to the products due to the high costs, then the populations and research subjects from developing contexts are exploited. Wenner's (2015, 77) account similarly makes this clear-cut connection between the social requirement and exploitation: the argument is that researchers and sponsors commit a moral wrong, namely exploitation, when a particular research project has no value for a host community. I will furthermore refer to this as the *Exploitation Argument*.

To prevent exploitation, research needs to generate socially valuable information tailored to the health needs of the respective LMIC communities. The argument relies on the assumption that host communities are *relevant stakeholders* who must partake in the fruits of research. As we have seen, Varmus and Satcher (1997) thought that placebo-controlled trials could be ethically justified as long as they would produce relevant information for countries. Glantz et al. (1998) argued that the intervention would need to be affordable and that there would need to be a realistic plan for funding the implementation of the intervention to avoid exploitation. In subsequent work, Emanuel and colleagues (2004, 930) suggested that the risk of exploitation in LMIC communities could be minimized when arrangements would be made to provide infrastructure that translates research results into health care practices for the benefit of the larger population.

The Missing Piece in the Debate: "Community Exploitation" and "the Social Value Requirement"

There are good reasons to cast doubt on the consistency of the concept of exploitation as applied to communities, which has a direct impact on the consistency of the Exploitation Argument, that is, exploitation framed as an insufficient knowledge gain for communities.

"Community Exploitation" within a Transactional Theory of Exploitation

A rigorous conception of community exploitation has never been developed in the literature concerning the fair treatment of host communities, starting from the early work by Glantz et al. (1998) and Annas and Grodin (1998). Hitherto, the debate on exploitation in health research has for the most part focused on the exploitation of *individual research subjects*, not *communities* (Malmqvist 2013, 2017; Wertheimer 1999, 2011; Wenner 2018b).

According to many commentators (Hawkins and Emanuel 2008, chap. 2; Malmqvist 2013; Resnik 2003), Allan Wertheimer has offered the most comprehensive, practical, and in-depth account of exploitation in health research. Since I will explain his approach in more detail in the next chapter, let me just note for now that Wertheimer (1999, 2011) offers a model of exploitation on which one party A exploits another party B by "taking unfair advantage." He furthermore defines "taking unfair advantage" as unfair distribution of benefits and burdens in a transaction between A and B. This is widely known as the "transactional fairness" or "transaction-specific" account of exploitation (Malmqvist and Szigeti 2019; Wenner 2018b).[2] It is noteworthy that the current discussion about fair benefit-sharing and exploitation of host communities among contemporary research ethicists has almost exclusively taken place within the limits of Wertheimer's transaction-specific theory of exploitation (Emanuel et al. 2004, 2008; Wendler and Rid 2017; Wenner 2018a). But Wertheimer's (1999, 2011) highly acclaimed transaction-specific account of exploitation has never been convincingly applied to *communities* in the context of health research.[3] Yet, a robust concept of what I will call from now on "community exploitation" is a theoretical void in the debate on the fair treatment of host communities.

Community Exploitation and the Social Value Requirement Revisited

While earlier discussions focused on the content of the social value requirement, more recent work has been directed toward its justification (Holzer 2017; London 2012; Resnik 2016; Wendler and Rid 2017; Wenner 2018a). Glantz et al. (1998) as well as Annas and Grodin (1998) appeal to a perfect symmetry between community exploitation and the social value requirement. Exploitation occurs when developed countries benefit from clinical trials and the underdeveloped countries that host those trials cannot "possibly derive information [from the trial] that would be of any benefit to its population" (Glantz 1998, 3, see Table 2.1). Thus, avoiding exploitation of communities entails that a research project ought to aim for the creation of valuable information or socially valuable knowledge for communities. But then, the social value requirement can be questioned on the same grounds as community exploitation: the main critique concerns the use of a transaction-specific account of exploitation to justify a requirement that primarily affects host communities and not transacting partners (Wenner 2018b).

We may reframe the conceptual problem related to that in the following way: the social value requirement seems to serve as a safeguard against community exploitation. Any research trial should avoid the moral wrong of community exploitation: research morally ought to seek social value for communities. However, considering it from the transactional viewpoint, exploitation cannot possibly apply to community members who are part of the broader background context of transactions, as these do not participate in an exploitative "transaction" with researchers and sponsors (Wenner 2018b, 569).

But there seems to be a way out. As Emanuel et al. (2000, 2004) suggest, the social value of research serves as a safeguard against the exploitation of individual *research participants*, not *community members* other than research participants (see Wendler and Rid 2017). I will call this argument by Emanuel and colleagues' (2004, 930) the *No Good Reason Argument*. This argument attempts to establish a different link between exploitation and the social value requirement. Exposing research subjects to risks without aiming for socially valuable knowledge is exploitative because such studies use research subjects "for no good reason" (Emanuel et al. 2000, 2703; Hughes 2012).

However, Wertheimer (2015) strictly denies the relation between exploitation and the social value of knowledge, as follows. In his paper "The Social Value Requirement Reconsidered," Wertheimer (2015) generally considers the social value requirement as neither necessary nor sufficient to avoid the exploitation of individual research participants. Individual research subjects are not less or more exploited when research yields social value, interpreted as a potential benefit that accrues to a local host community or society, as it is only ethical to expose research subjects to risks and burdens independently of the social value research produces. The social value is not sufficient to protect participants from exploitation because *participants* may be entitled to some fair level of benefits even if a trial yields social value more broadly (Wenner 2018a). Otherwise, the beneficiaries in society exploitatively free-ride on the research subjects who participate and accept risks for the good of society. Indeed, exploitation would then be even more likely because individual risks are taken to be balanced out by broader social benefits.

Furthermore, the social value requirement is not a necessary condition for preventing exploitation of research subjects. If there are no risks for research subjects or if the individual risks are outweighed by expected individual benefits or even a monetary compensation to the research subjects, the social value is not necessary. Roughly speaking, Wertheimer argues that if they are rational agents, individuals care about their own net benefit in trials. He argues that in research without individual therapeutic benefits, subjects can reasonably accept financial or other benefits (e.g., collaborating with a good cause) for their participation that exceed the risks of participation (Wertheimer 2015, 304–5). He thus segregates individual benefits and risks from the general social benefits of research. For these reasons, Wertheimer (2015) thinks that Emanuel et al.'s No Good Reason Argument cannot serve as a sound justification for the social value requirement.

In my view, Wertheimer has rightly pointed to the persistent weaknesses, mostly the lack of conceptual backing for certain concepts in current widely used research ethics frameworks. Admittedly, there have been other attempts to rescue the social value requirement, mostly unrelated to the Exploitation Argument.[4] Wendler and Rid (2017) have offered a multifaceted account of possible justifications for the social value of research. Wenner (2018a) has argued that we need to abandon the transactional model that has been unquestioned ever since Wertheimer's view began dominating the literature related to exploitation in health research. Following Wenner, I believe that this is perhaps the most promising road to take if we want to, first, make sense of the Exploitation Argument and, second, take the interests of host communities as stakeholders seriously.

Road Ahead: Accounting for Fair Benefits, Community Exploitation, and the Social Value Requirement

This chapter has so far presented the more general lines of argument in the form of a historical reconstruction of an ongoing debate in research ethics. The further approach will be to show that a modification of the Exploitation Argument and a proper framework of "community exploitation" outside the transactional paradigm allow us to develop a valuable theory of fair benefit-sharing.

Accounting for "Community Exploitation"

There are good reasons for developing a sound concept of community exploitation. First, I see my own conceptual elaborations as an interpretation of what has been theorized in the traditional research ethics literature over the last three decades. Offering a framework for community exploitation would be in line with the tradition of research ethics, that is, research ethics as it has been practiced among academics since the 1990s. Many scholars, apart from Wertheimer, implicitly or explicitly assume that host communities are exploited if they do not receive an adequate share of the benefits from a research enterprise. My aim, therefore, is to enrich existing concepts in the research ethics literature rather than to overturn a whole set of theories and concepts.

Second, beyond this pragmatic argument, there is a substantive argument for an enriched conception of community exploitation. Scholars still working within the transactional model should find new ways to explain why members of a community are stakeholders in a transaction that supposedly happens between a private corporation and those who should be compensated for their direct participation in the transaction (i.e., research subjects) (Wenner 2018a). What scholars tend to forget are nontransactional contributions that set up the background conditions for a successful research enterprise (see Chapter 4).

Third, there is another sort of moral argument the transactional account of exploitation fails to address. Wertheimer's theory of exploitation remains silent regarding structural deficits or "background injustices" researchers take advantage of, a recurrent concern in the literature on research in LMICs (Malmqvist 2013, 2017; Petryna 2009; Wenner 2016; see Chapters 3 and 6). It seems worthwhile to elaborate more on the immediate connection between structural injustices leading to poverty and powerlessness in LMICs and the propensity of host countries to agree to exploitative research studies. Structural conditions matter to exploitation when foreign corporations take advantage of injustice, which is not questioned in the transactional paradigm (see

Malmqvist 2013, 2017, Macklin 2004). Structural deficits, including poverty, powerlessness, and economic dependency, are often identified as major driving forces behind exploitative clinical trials (see Malmqvist 2017; Petryna 2009). Also, structural injustices seem to be important in another respect, which complements Wertheimer's (2015) concern that the social value requirement cannot protect research subjects from exploitation. The exploitation of individuals, e.g., of research subjects, can persist and be perpetuated even if a host community benefits greatly and sufficiently from research. This is true when benefits are very unequally distributed among community members, a concern related to structural factors (Wenner 2018b).

The following chapters will address all these points. One aim is to come up with a new interpretation of "community exploitation" that leaves the transaction-specific model behind. A more appropriate conceptual framework for community exploitation is needed to make headway in the current debates. Moreover, I want to address the relation between structural injustice and exploitation, which is a major issue in the context of research in LMICs. The insights gained through structural accounts of exploitation may be helpful in such discussions because the current predominating framework of transaction-specific fairness is limited in accounting for this moral dimension.

Making Sense of the Social Value Requirement

I believe many of us have the strong intuition that it is unjust or exploitative when the benefits of research almost exclusively accrue to researchers and sponsors as well as citizens from HICs who are in possession of the resources to effectively implement and use the drugs tested in LMICs. In the case scenarios discussed in the introductory chapter, one suspects that host communities reap an unfairly small portion of the benefits.

But working within the transactional paradigm does not justify the social value requirement, at least on the grounds of exploitation. As previously stated, I mainly seek to offer a new justification for fair benefit-sharing and a new conceptualization of community exploitation. This constitutes a new interpretation of both the social value requirement and the exploitation argument.

Concluding Remarks

While early commentators in the 1990s were mostly concerned about the "double standard" of clinical trials in LMIC contexts, later debate from the early 2000s shifted toward the exploitation argument and the social value requirement, based on the premise that offshored research in LMICs should fairly benefit local host communities.

To this day, many authors conceptualize "community exploitation" and the "social value requirement" within Wertheimer's transactional account. This has led to unsatisfactory positions regarding the conceptualization of obligations owed to host communities. A sound and comprehensive account of community exploitation and fair benefit-sharing remains a conceptual gap in the current research ethics literature to date. The following chapters are devoted to providing a workable interpretation and a sound philosophical basis for these concepts.

3

Transactional Models for Fair Benefit-Sharing: Three Fundamental Objections

Toward "Transactional Models" of Fair Benefit-Sharing

I concluded the previous chapter by explaining that Wertheimer's transactional stance does not suit the purposes of justifying fair benefit-sharing with host communities. I argued that the transactional argument neither accounts for the social value requirement—the idea that socially valuable knowledge should accrue to host communities—nor acknowledges that communities can be exploited. I now reframe the chronological narrative of the past chapter more analytically by introducing two what I previously called "normative models." I argue that the debate in the literature has given rise to two major transactional models, both of which have been defended in the field of international health research ethics. I will refer to these models as the *vulnerability model* and the *economic model* (Wertheimer 2011) that is best known in research ethics as the *fair benefits approach* (Emanuel and Participants 2008; Participants 2004; Schulz-Baldes et al. 2007). The label "transactional" is owed to the fact that these models do *not* formulate obligations that find expression in cooperative schemes, as in (for instance) a basic structure (Wenner 2018a).[1] Transactional models are nonpolitical in the sense that they establish obligations between individual agents irrespective of their wider cooperative or institutional relationships.[2]

The *vulnerability model* takes up the basic ethical requirements of responsiveness to communities' health needs and priorities (CIOMS-WHO 2002, 2016; Homedes y Ugalde 2015; London 2008; Macklin 2004a,b; Pratt and Hyder 2015) and reasonable availability (CIOMS-WHO 2002, guideline 10) or post-trial availability (CIOMS-WHO 2016, guideline 2) of knowledge and interventions that are proven to be effective during the course of a research trial (Crouch and Arras 1998; Glantz et al. 1998; Homedes y Ugalde 2015; Macklin 2004a,b; WMA 2013).[3] These requirements have been widely acknowledged in international research guidelines, such as the CIOMS-WHO guidelines (2016), and, notably, address the general concern and the increasing recognition that LMIC communities in low-resource settings do not adequately benefit from research outputs (CIOMS-WHO 2016, guideline 2; Pratt and Loff 2014). The second model I would like to introduce is the "fair benefits approach" (Emanuel et al. 2008); I will call it the *economic model*.[4] The fair benefits approach is perhaps the most-cited and best-developed model in the research ethics literature. It has emerged as a critical answer to the criteria of responsiveness and reasonable availability and offers an alternative solution to the fair treatment of host communities in international health research.

As outlined in the introduction, any normative (transactional or political) model specific to my research area ought to address the following questions:

i. Do researchers and sponsors bear obligations toward host communities? (Justification requirement); and
ii. If this is the case, what is the content of these obligations? (Content requirement)

In what follows, I will show how both the vulnerability and the economic model relate to the justification and content requirements. Further, I will formulate three fundamental critiques pointing to the weaknesses both transactional models show in this respect. First, I argue that they fall short of providing a sound justification for fair benefit-sharing, as they fail to include satisfying obligations toward host communities. This problem is notably grounded in a flawed transactional conception of community exploitation (see Chapter 2). Second, I argue that transactional models insufficiently address background injustices. Third, I will criticize the procedural framework offered by the economic model to determine what "fair benefits" are. Pointing to the problems of these transactional models allows me to better carve out the advantages of a political (nontransactional) model in the next chapters.

The Vulnerability Model

The vulnerability model[5] consists of two ethical requirements to characterize fair benefits: responsiveness of research to health needs and priorities, and reasonable or post-trial availability of knowledge and the tested drugs. As I will argue, the vulnerability model does not deliver a sophisticated foundation to establish host communities as stakeholders with a right to fair benefits and researchers and sponsors as the corresponding obligation bearers. However, both requirements deserve a place of honor in the discussion because they have been among the first accounts to address the moral claims of communities. Here, it is important to mention that both requirements are direct responses to the concern of what is commonly known as "safari" or "helicopter" research in the literature. The main underlying narrative is that researchers and sponsors from rich nations conduct trials in developing countries and free themselves from any further obligations to address a community's interests once they obtain the desired data (Macklin 2011). Some scholars complained that developing countries are used as mere "biological resources" for the testing of drugs that eventually benefit the global rich (Sethuraman 2001). This narrative is echoed in one of the comments on the mother-to-child HIV transmission studies presented by the US National Bioethics Advisory Commission (NBAC) in the 2001 report *Ethical and Policy Issues in International Research: Clinical Trials in Developing Countries*:

> Pharmaceutical industry puts pressure on researchers to conduct research on their drugs and we are acting as guinea pigs for the first world. This industry is actively participating in unethical research which could never be carried out in other developed countries or the United States. Some felt that the United States did nothing to stop unethical research even when it was aware that it was taking place. (NBAC 2001a, B-90)

As I argued in Chapter 2, research ethicists since the 1990s have characterized research with an insufficient social value for host communities as exploitative enterprises (Glantz et al. 1998). The ethical requirements of responsiveness to health needs and priorities as well as reasonable availability of knowledge and tested drugs emerged in the historical discussion initiated by Annas and

Grodin (1998), Glantz et al. (1998), and Macklin (2004a,b) and have been widely defended in the literature of health research ethics ever since (Homedes y Ugalde 2016; London 2008; Pratt and Hyder 2014; Wenner 2017). Nowadays the responsiveness requirement is complemented by the requirement of reasonable availability of knowledge and tested drugs.

Both requirements are constituent components of important current international ethics guidelines for health-related research (CIOMS-WHO 2016; WMA 2013).[6] The Declaration of Helsinki's (WMA 2013) accounts as follows for "vulnerable" groups and individuals:

> Medical research with a vulnerable group is only justified if the research is responsive to the health needs or priorities of this group and the research cannot be carried out in a non-vulnerable group. In addition, this group should stand to benefit from the knowledge, practices or interventions that result from the research. (WMA 2013, paragraph 20)

The Declaration of Helsinki (WMA 2013) makes salient the fact that the two ethical requirements—responsiveness and reasonable availability—specifically apply to "vulnerable" groups, which does not necessarily hold for populations that are not vulnerable or disadvantaged (Macklin 2011). Here, I avoid arguing why "vulnerable" groups should be considered as such and instead adhere to a minimal notion that populations lack substantive capacities to having the means of "fully protect their own interests." Applied to the context of my research question, it suffices to assume that LMIC populations in low-resource settings can be *prima facie* reasonably considered vulnerable.[7]

Responsiveness of Research to Health Needs or Priorities

Responsiveness is an ethical requirement intended to ensure that the limited resources in international research are directed to health problems that are actually of concern or burdensome in the host communities. The CIOMS-WHO (2016) guidelines acknowledge this as follows:

> Before instituting a plan to undertake research in a population or community with limited resources or infrastructure, the sponsor, researchers, and

> relevant public health authority must ensure that the research is responsive to the health needs or priorities of the communities or populations where the research will be conducted. (CIOMS-WHO 2016, guideline 2)

Together with the local health institutions of LMICs, international researchers and sponsors are required to provide host populations with the opportunity to benefit from externally funded research. Guideline 2 (CIOMS-WHO 2016) specifies that being responsive to health needs means seeking and providing research outputs that are socially valuable to the host community. However, responsiveness alone cannot ensure that health benefits accrue to them. This is the case because interventions proven effective must also be made available in the communities (CIOMS-WHO 2002, guideline 10).

Furthermore, responsiveness is typically defined as the alignment of research with the *health needs* and/or *health priorities* of a host community or country. The conception of responsiveness of research to health needs focuses on any health condition or disease prevalent in the community. Responsiveness to a health priority, in turn, does not necessarily coincide with every health need because it is restricted to health conditions that are considered most pressing in a country (London 2008; Millum 2012; Pratt and Hyder 2014).

Availability of Interventions and Knowledge

Reasonable availability (CIOMS-WHO 2002) or *post-trial availability* (CIOMS-WHO 2016) is the second ethical requirement of the vulnerability model and closely related to the responsiveness requirement. Likewise, it is acknowledged in guideline 2 of the latest CIOMS-WHO (2016) version:

> As part of their obligation, sponsors, researchers must also make every effort in cooperation with government and civil society to make available as soon as possible any intervention or product developed, and/or knowledge generated, for the population or community in which the research is carried out. (CIOMS-WHO 2016, guideline 2)

As the CIOMS-WHO (2016) guidelines state, it is not sufficient to adhere to the responsiveness requirement in order to put to rest concerns about "safari" research where researchers and sponsors collect valuable data without appropriately benefiting host societies. Rather, the ethical requirement of responsiveness goes along with the requirement of reasonable or post-trial availability, meaning that if an intervention, drug, or other innovation turns out to be successful and beneficial, researchers and sponsors should help make both the generated knowledge and the intervention available to research subjects and the host community (Crouch and Arras 1998; Glantz et al. 1998).

The comment on guideline 2 states that stakeholders in charge of guaranteeing the requirements must determine their scope and application in practice on a case-by-case basis (see also comment on guideline 10, CIOMS-WHO 2002). This evaluation should address the time for which the intervention or product is developed, benefits to research subjects and to the population, the severity of subjects' medical condition and the costs.

The Normative Justification of the Vulnerability Model

Neither the Declaration of Helsinki nor the CIOMS-WHO guidelines specifically state an ethical justification for the responsiveness and availability requirements. Nevertheless, it seems that there are two candidates for such a justification: the social value requirement and the concept of exploitation of the vulnerable.

Regarding the first option: the social value of research (i.e., the knowledge and potential health gain generated through the research process) underpins the establishment of the responsiveness and availability requirements. The CIOMS-WHO guidelines (2016, comment on guideline 2) support this view by stating that research seeking to provide social value manifests itself "automatically" in responsiveness to significant health needs and/or priorities present in a host community or population. Responsiveness to health needs and priorities together with the aim to make the tested intervention available reflect the goal of attaining the greatest possible social value from research.

After the revision of the 2016 CIOMS guidelines, Wenner (2017) has not only tried to assess the social value criterion, but also demonstrated how this framework can be used to inform the responsiveness requirement. She argues that given the social investments of physical and human capital and the opportunity costs associated with biomedical research, the social value of research ought to be an ethical guiding principle for research projects. The social value framework can function at the global level to inform judgments about what ultimately constitutes the motivations behind responsiveness. If trials leave unaddressed concerns of host communities where drugs are tested, those communities bear a disproportionate share of the burdens while reaping only few long-term gains from the socially valuable research output (Wenner 2017, 101). Thus, given that the epistemic output of a project is not responsive to local health needs in the short term, it is unlikely that locally valuable knowledge is ever generated and there should be a presumption against the conduct of research that a priori fails to meet responsiveness (Wenner 2017, 104).

Wenner's (2017) concern is that a "broad" interpretation of the social value requirement—holding that research generally needs to aim at sufficient social value and that this includes basic research—is not enough (see Wendler and Rid 2017). We ought to adhere to a more demanding, "narrow" interpretation of the social value requirement in LMIC contexts, namely, that research produces a *significant* epistemic output for a host community. While the social value of research is a general guiding principle for any health-related research enterprise and is not specific to research conducted in LMIC contexts (Emanuel et al. 2000), the comment on guideline 2 (CIOMS-WHO 2016) specifies that offshored research that does not yield *significant* fruits for the health improvement or knowledge gain in LMICs is unethical. Therefore, preliminary research in early phases without a workable drug as its end goal may only be allowed in exceptional cases, for instance, if research studies cannot be carried out in more developed countries. This is, again, the core of the vulnerability model: choosing "vulnerable" groups comes along with more demanding ethical obligations on the part of researchers and sponsors.

Yet, the specifications of guideline 2 (CIOMS-WHO 2016) already point to another, perhaps more fundamental justification for responsiveness and reasonable availability: on this view, the requirements are designed to prevent vulnerable communities with less bargaining power than international researchers and sponsors from exploitation (CIOMS-WHO 2002). The connection seems clear. As I explained in the last chapter, a framework for the fair treatment of host communities bears comparison with the criterion requiring socially valuable outcomes of research for communities. In turn, socially valuable knowledge under the vulnerability model is guaranteed by the responsiveness and the reasonable availability requirements. By making socially valuable research available to LMIC communities through the establishment of the two requirements, researchers and sponsors prevent the most vulnerable parties in a research project from being exploited.

But what does that mean? I previously claimed that a defensible criterion explaining when individuals or communities are exploited is missing. However, an intuitive definition of exploitation clearly appeals to the idea that exploitation is conceptually related to the vulnerability of individuals and populations. LMIC communities can be vulnerable when they are powerless, poor, and often dependent of the goodwill of the affluent. The two ethical requirements seem to be compelling safeguards for the ethical conduct of research in "vulnerable" populations where governments often lack the means or infrastructure to investigate ethical breaches and to make medical products widely available (CIOMS-WHO, comment on guideline 2).

The Economic Model

The economic model, most widely known as the fair benefits approach, is probably the most comprehensive transactional model developed for fair benefit-sharing in international health research. Since the economic model will be the focal point of my critique in this chapter, it deserves a brief introduction.

Most of the early debates in international research ethics were based on the vulnerability model, i.e., the responsiveness and availability requirements (CIOMS-WHO 1993; CIOMS-WHO 2002; Crouch and Arras 1998; Glantz et al. 1998). And still, the vulnerability model has not vanished from notice in international guideline documents (CIOMS-WHO 2016; WMA 2013). However, an international working group convened in 2001 by the US National Institutes of Health criticized the two requirements for being too conceptually narrow and misleading (Emanuel and Participants 2008; Participants 2004; Schulz-Baldes et al. 2007). The group subsequently proposed a broader framework, the fair benefits approach, to account for collateral benefits outside the focus of the two ethical requirements; these benefits included health services, public-health measures, employments and economic activity, capacity-building, and financial rewards (Schulz-Baldes et al. 2007).

Regarding the critique of the two requirement, various scholars—including the Participants in the 2001 Conference on Ethical Aspects of Research in Developing Countries (Participants 2004), Wolitz et al. (2009), Emanuel (2008), Emanuel and Participants (2008), and Millum (2012)—think that the vulnerability model shows some substantial weaknesses. Most notably, the responsiveness and reasonable availability requirements fail to address the *level* of benefits a community must receive. To put it another way, even if research is responsive and made available to communities, one cannot necessarily protect LMIC communities from exploitation (Emanuel 2008).

According to Emanuel (2008), individual research subjects and host populations are exploited when they receive an unfairly small share of benefits generated through research, or bear disproportionally high burdens in comparison to researchers and sponsors, such as the pharmaceutical industry (Ballantyne 2010a; Emanuel 2008; Emanuel and Participants 2008). Here, exploitation reflects a state in which the distribution of a surplus value in a cooperative transaction is unfair. Recall that I reconstructed the vulnerability model so as to relate its ethical justification to the social value requirement and the exploitation of the vulnerable. The vulnerability model, however, does not interpret community exploitation in terms of an unfair *distribution* of benefits and burdens.[8]

The economic model provides additional arguments for why the vulnerability model fails (see Emanuel and Participants 2008), from which I choose four important objections (see Table 3.1). First, the strict interpretation of the social value requirement as a quest for responsiveness (Wenner 2017) and reasonable availability may serve as a general guiding principle *prima facie*, but it is not specific to a particular research context. There may be other substantial benefits, such as the overall improvement of care facilities and infrastructure, that could justify a clinical trial even though the study is unresponsive to health needs and priorities or does not meet the demand for reasonable availability (Emanuel and Participants 2008, 295).

Second, even though the responsiveness and reasonable availability requirements can help realize the preferences of developing countries as well as foreground the aim of addressing diseases of the global poor more effectively, the requirements would seem to lead to a potentially dangerous "all-or-nothing" game. Defenders of the economic model assume that countries cannot choose between a responsive study and an unresponsive study, but solely between a study (responsive or not) and no study at all. In this scenario, the responsiveness and reasonable availability requirements may oblige developing countries to forgo research that would have otherwise been beneficial (Wolitz et al. 2009), and moreover may hamper the autonomous decisions by communities about what benefits are worth the risks of a research trial. Neglect can be worse than exploitative research conditions (Emanuel and Participants 2008; Rivera Lopez 2017).

Third, Emanuel and Participants (2008, 297) believe that even late phase clinical studies provide very uncertain benefits to populations regarding the reasonable availability of the tested interventions, as the requirement depends on whether a new medical intervention is successful in its test. If there is true clinical equipoise[9] at the beginning of a Phase 3 trial, the success of the intervention to be tested should not yet be determined.

Forth, Emanuel and Participants (2008, 297–8) warn that the requirements of the vulnerability model can easily lead to "undue inducement," meaning that deprived populations enroll in excessively risky research to obtain promised health benefits.[10]

There are several lines of argument available to counter these critiques (Table 3.1). Macklin (2004a,b), whom I interpret as one of the core defenders of the vulnerability model, counters that the requirements can neither avoid exploitation nor offer a precise allocation mechanism to determine how much of the generated benefits should accrue to LMIC communities. Nevertheless, the requirements are necessary (but not sufficient) to avoid exploitation in health research. Millum (2012) adds to this rationale that responsiveness and availability serve as heuristic tools to obtain a fair distribution of benefits. Fulfilling the ethical requirements means probably coming close to what we would call a "fair" distribution of benefits.

Table 3.1 The Vulnerability Model: Features, Objections from the Economic Model and Replies. *See Wendler and Shah (2017)*

Model Feature	Objection	Reply
Fair Distribution and Exploitation	No criterion or procedural mechanism for determining whether a distribution is "fair"	Requirements are "heuristic tools" to attain an approximately fair distribution (Millum 2012)
"All or Nothing Game"	The two requirements, responsiveness and availability, can be too restrictive in the sense that foreign researchers and sponsors are discouraged from conducting a clinical study; this is worse for the community than an unresponsive study	
Reasonable Availability	Under true equipoise, there is a high risk that the tested medicine will not be made available	Frequently, the success of the intervention is *ex ante* very likely (Glantz et al. 1998; Lurie and Wolfe 1997)
Undue Inducement	Populations may agree to unreasonably risky research because of expected health benefits	Undue inducement is a problem that applies to any sort of benefit (Ledford 2014)
Social Value Requirement	The social value is not only expressed in the responsiveness and availability requirements	The requirements are necessary, not sufficient (Macklin 2004a, 2004b)

Furthermore, we should not forget that the designs of many clinical trials under a "double standard" (e.g., the HIV transmission studies in the 1990s) do not necessarily adhere to strict equipoise, meaning that the placebo treatment arm is *ex ante* worse off than the active arm, precisely when the effect of the drug seems likely to be positive (Glantz et al. 1998; Lurie and Wolfe 1997). Finally, regarding the fourth objection put forward by the defenders of the economic model, it does not seem clear why undue inducement would solely apply to the promise of reasonable availability, but not to other sorts of benefits such as capacity-building, training, and education. Direct investments and monetary benefits seem especially likely to produce undue incentives to participate in risky research or to breach standard ethical norms. For example, Jeff Blackmer, executive director of the Canadian Medical Association's ethics office and member of the 2013 World Medical Association's Ethics Committee, explained that there is evidence in the history of international health research that some community leaders were pressuring locals to enroll in clinical trials in order to secure the facilities, like schools or clean water projects, that came along as benefits of participation in research projects (Ledford 2014). Therefore, the World Medical Association (2013) deleted such provisions in the last revision of the Declaration of Helsinki.

Despite these arguments, proponents of the economic model may be right in saying that researchers and sponsors sometimes owe additional benefits to a host population beyond the requirements of the vulnerability model. Such benefits may include the improvement of the health infrastructure, training for laboratory personnel and health workers, education of the public about the nature of research, and education regarding the benefits likely to result from the particular study in question. While capacity-building should be an established component of any research project conducted in low-resource settings, other types of benefits depend on the circumstances of a clinical study and the specific terms of the collaboration among researchers, sponsors, local health authorities, and communities.

For instance, by pointing to the distribution of benefits, Emanuel and Participants (2008) explain that the Havrix trial is harder to analyze than the vulnerability model suggests (see Chapter 1). The requirements of responsiveness and reasonable availability were clearly not fulfilled in the Havrix trial: there was no systematic plan to incorporate the tested hepatitis A vaccine into the Thai national health plan; in addition, hepatitis A was not a pressing health concern, as many people had previously been immunized. However, the economic model argues that other compensating benefits were offered to the host community: among others, a hepatitis B vaccine for participants and health workers, the improvement of infrastructure, training of health personnel, and public education.

I contend that the objections to the vulnerability model seem compelling in some but not all respects. Here, it is certainly true that the vulnerability model fails to offer an account for the fair *distribution* of benefits. I argued that any normative model for fair benefit-sharing does not only need to address (i) the justification requirement (i.e., how obligations to host communities can be grounded) but also (ii) the content requirement. The vulnerability model provides us with two content requirements to characterize fair benefits, namely, responsiveness to health needs and priorities and reasonable availability of the tested intervention and knowledge. However, it is true that the model does not offer a principle able to determine what a "fair share" of this content, i.e., the socially valuable research output, is. It is true that fair shares can be fixed in prior agreements, but the responsiveness and availability requirements do not provide us with a general criterion for determining fair benefits or a justification of the same. Since I interpret the fair treatment of host communities in terms of host communities' claim to *distributive fairness* (Chapter 1), I conclude that the economic model might be a valuable alternative to the vulnerability model, at least at first glance.

Fair Benefit-sharing

The defenders of the economic model offer an alternative approach to the vulnerability model based on a *transaction-specific* conception of exploitation (Emanuel et al. 2004; Emanuel and Participants 2008; Participants 2004; Wendler and Shah 2017). The rationale behind this is to establish a criterion of exploitation to evaluate whether a research study complies with fair terms of cooperation. Emanuel (2008, 726) calls the fair benefits approach the "most developed and detailed alternative" to the reasonable availability and responsiveness requirements (Emanuel 2008; Millum 2012). The fair benefits framework entered the CIOMS-WHO guidelines in 2016; the guidelines stipulate that "[s]ponsors, researchers, governmental authorities, and research ethics committees must ensure that the benefits and burdens of research are equitably distributed" (CIOMS-WHO 2016, guideline 3).

The fair benefits approach consists of three principles: *fair benefits*, *collaborative partnerships*, and *transparency*. All are meant to ensure that the terms of a transaction are fair. While collaborative partnerships and transparency focus on the procedural mechanisms needed to attain a fair distribution of benefits and community involvement,[11] the principle of fair benefits specifies the "benefits" at stake. A fair distribution of benefits implies that benefits must increase with burdens, with benefits to others, and with larger relative contributions to the scheme in question (Gbadegesin and Wendler 2006; London 2008; London and Zollman 2010; Participants 2004, 22). According to Emanuel (2008), benefits can be of various types: benefits to research participants during the research, benefits to the population during the research, and benefits to the participants and/or population after the completion of research.

Importantly, other than the responsiveness and reasonable availability requirements, the fair benefits framework does not give explicit guidance on the specific content of agreements researchers and sponsors ought to adhere to. Proponents of the fair benefits approach only state that benefits and burdens must be *shared fairly* among all stakeholders. Nevertheless, the economic model meets the content requirement in the sense that *any* benefit is considered to be morally legitimate as long as the sum of benefits received constitutes a *fair share* of the overall benefits and as long as communities participate in fair negotiations to determine the content of the same.

The Justification of the Economic Model

The fair benefits approach (or economic model) grounds its normative concept of fair benefit-sharing in the exploitation argument. Exploitation, or "taking unfair advantage" of another party, is an evil everyone should avoid in health research. According to its defenders, the fair benefits approach grew out of a specific account of transaction-specific exploitation based on Wertheimer's (1999, 2011) theory of exploitation (Emanuel and Participants 2008; Emanuel 2008). Transaction-specific exploitation occurs when an unfair distribution of benefits and burdens is generated through a mutual transaction (Emanuel and Participants 2008; Gbadegesin and Wendler 2006; Wertheimer 1999). A transaction between two parties A and B (individuals or groups) involves exploitation of A when

> 1) *B*, or some third party benefits from *A*'s involvement in the transaction; and 2) *A* receives an unfair level of benefits as a result of its involvement in the transaction. Whether the benefits a party receives as a result of its engagement in a transaction are *fair* depends on the burdens that the transaction places on that party. As party *A* bears greater burdens—increased risks, inconveniences, costs, harms, discomfort—*A* should receive greater benefits to ensure a fair transaction. Whether a party's level of benefits is fair also depends on the level of benefits that others receive as a result of the party's efforts in the transaction. As party *A*'s efforts produce more benefit for *B*, *A* should receive greater benefits to ensure a fair transaction. (Gbadegesin and Wendler 2006, 249, emphasis present in the original text)

The crucial point is that exploitation occurs when B[12] or a third party "takes unfair advantage" of another party A. Importantly, even if both parties *consent to* and/or *benefit from* an interaction, exploitation can still occur; this is then called "mutually advantageous" and "consensual" exploitation (Wertheimer 1999).

Emanuel and Participants (2008, 292f) state that exploitation takes place on a "micro" level, meaning that the concept is about harms from discrete interactions, rather than about the larger social justice of the distribution of background rights and resources (2008, 293). In their view, what they call "Rawlsian" fairness, or principles regulating a "basic structure,"[13] exceed the transactional level. This means constitutional arrangements, taxes, and fair opportunities are *wrongly* applied to the context of micro-level decisions (Emanuel and participants 2008, 294). In order to get a better grasp of what an unfair transaction *within a mutually advantageous and consensual exploitation* entails, we need to have a closer look at Wertheimer's (1999) theory of exploitation, which the defenders of the economic model rely on.

Wertheimer's Theory of Transaction-Specific Exploitation

In chapter 7 of his book *Exploitation*, Wertheimer (1999) develops a theory of exploitation that elaborates the conditions of "unfair" or "exploitative" transactions. He distinguishes among several types of exploitation between a potential exploiter A and an exploitee B, among them, harmful exploitation and mutually advantageous exploitation. Wertheimer furthermore defines two dimensions of a transaction: (1) the benefit to A, which is relevant to both harmful and mutually advantageous exploitation; and (2) the fairness of the transaction to B, which is the central concern of mutually advantageous exploitation. When Wertheimer refers to the fairness of a transaction (the dimension of greatest interest to me), he is not referring to the background fairness but to transaction-specific fairness. According to this account, in cases where A's status is superior to B's, one needs to distinguish between fairness as a principle for the distribution of social resources and fairness as a principle for transactions. Wertheimer's conception of exploitation is grounded in a transaction-specific principle of fairness that determines the moral legitimacy of a transaction.

Furthermore, Wertheimer investigates different distribution principles or mechanisms according to which benefits (and burdens) may be shared between A and B, including rational bargaining, equality, the contribution principle, and fair hypothetical markets. Regarding the latter, Wertheimer (1999, 230) identifies a principle capable of providing a plausible conception of a fair transaction for a wide range of cases. The "fair market value" is a hypothetical or counterfactual concept, which represents the price an informed and unpressured seller would receive from an informed and unpressured buyer if a commodity were sold on the market. Given the history of the concept of justice, Wertheimer's fair market value interpretation appeals to what Henry Sidgwick (1907, 289) calls the "individualistic ideal" of justice. The "individualistic ideal" means that choices are made by individuals. Market efficiency through methodological individualism under the assumptions of the absence of market distortions implies that transactions yield fair outcomes.

Wertheimer (1999, 231) appeals to the reader's intuition with the analogy that a fair exchange of goods, including services, would result among friends who are willing to commit to a fair exchange. The fair market value would then be on a par with an amicable exchange. In this condition, fairness also appeals to nondiscrimination, disallowing alteration of the terms of exchange because of gender, religion, race, or arbitrary reasons. However, the competitive—here a synonym for *ideal*—market price does not reflect a "deep" principle[14] of justice. It may not be a "just price" all things considered, including initial distributive injustices prevalent in a bigger social scheme (see Roemer

1996). Nevertheless, argues Wertheimer, an ideal market price does reflect a crucial moral dimension of the relationship between two parties involved in a transaction.[15] The market price represents a nonexploitative price at which *neither party takes special unfair advantage* of particular defects in the other's decision-making capacity or her vulnerabilities (Wertheimer 1999, 232; see Gauthier 1986). Moreover, building on Wertheimer's principle, we may add that ideal (and thus perfectly competitive) markets are normatively attractive because they are efficient in the sense of being Pareto-optimal, meaning that it is impossible to reallocate resources and goods in a way so as to make any one individual or preference criterion better-off without making at least one other individual or preference criterion worse-off (Arneson 2008; Gauthier 1986).

Wertheimer's Theory of Exploitation Applied to International Health Research

Let us now return to exploitative practices in international health research. Interactions among researchers, sponsors, research subjects, and host communities are usually framed as mutually beneficial and consensual. We may suppose that research is *ex ante* expected to be beneficial to every participating party. I acknowledge that there may be problems related to voluntary consent in international health research. However, it is most interesting for my further normative analysis to deal with *mutually advantageous and consensual* transactions that are nonetheless exploitative in the sense that they result in an unfair distribution of the benefits and burdens generated in the transaction.

The economic model wants to establish an elaborate account providing us with an adequate normative justification for fair benefit-sharing with host communities. As Gbadegesin and Wendler (2006, 250) state, "whether a party's level of benefits is fair ... depends on the level of benefits that others receive as a result of the party's efforts in the transaction." Nevertheless, they do not offer a defensible criterion against which to assess whether benefits appropriately correspond to a party's contribution. We may, however, stick to some procedural criterion, like fair conditions of negotiation, in combination with Wertheimer's market criterion. Wertheimer himself investigates the possibility of applying his transaction-specific account of exploitation to the context of fair benefit-sharing in his chapter *Exploitation in Clinical Research* (2008) and his 2011 book *Rethinking the Ethics of Clinical Research*. Reframing the groundwork of the economic model, we can confirm that a community, B, is exploited when researchers and sponsors, A, give fewer benefits to B than are due to B according to the criterion of a "fair market price." Here, the economic model claims that researchers and sponsors have obligations that arise from their interaction with host communities (justification requirement; see Wertheimer 2011, 256). The content of such obligations is to offer host communities a fair market share of the benefits and burdens that occur in research (content requirement; see Emanuel and Participants 2008).

The two further pillars of the economic model—collaborative partnerships and transparency—are procedural mechanisms that shall guarantee that research results in fair negotiations and subsequently a fair division of benefits (see Emanuel 2008). Collaborative partnerships shall guarantee free and uncoerced decision-making by communities on, among other things, whether the benefits offered to participants and the community are sufficient. The principle of transparency would come along with a central repository of historical benefits agreements: an independent body that creates a publicly accessible repository of all formal and informal benefits agreements ever made (see Chapter 7). This would make it easier for host communities to assess what kind and quantity of benefits can be reasonably expected. Furthermore, transparency demands that community consultations are publicly held in forums that include representatives of the communities (Emanuel 2008, 725).

Three Objections against Transactional Models for Fair Benefit-Sharing

Various critiques have been brought against the vulnerability and the economic model (London and Zollman 2010; Schulz-Baldes et al. 2007; Wendler and Shah 2017).[16] I will present three substantive objections to the two most widely defended transactional models relevant to the fair treatment of host communities in international health research and corresponding ethics guidelines (see CIOMS-WHO 2016; WMA 2013). These objections concern first, the inability of transactional models to account for community exploitation; second, their failure to recognize background injustices; and third, the problem of imperfect markets. While I direct the first two objections to both the vulnerability and the economic model, my last critical point will address the faulty design of the economic model regarding its capacity to safeguard fair benefits. The three objections together show that the mainstream literature on fair benefit-sharing lacks a workable model.

First Objection: Transactional Models Fail to Account for Community Exploitation

Following the general outline of Chapter 2 and my previous comments in this chapter, I will show that the two transactional models first and foremost fail to account for community exploitation. Despite the fact that the vulnerability model has been, historically speaking, a valuable answer to cases of unethical clinical trials in the history of human health research, it yet lacks a framework that could possibly justify the responsiveness and the reasonable availability requirements at a more foundational level. The economic model seems to offer an account: transactional exploitation (Emanuel and Participants 2008). However, it remains unclear what kind of "transaction" or "interaction" we are talking about when basing "community exploitation" on a transaction-specific account.

The problem can be framed as follows. In analogy to an eye-opening example by Millum (2011, 250–1), when a street cleaner sweeps the ground and I benefit from that, I do not *per se* owe this worker any benefit in return that could be expressed as a special obligation of fairness. This directly relates to Wertheimer's (1999, 2011) transaction-specific account of fairness and exploitation, in which special fairness obligations toward the street cleaner would only arise if I were actively engaged in a mutual *transaction* with her (e.g., if we had made the deal that she would sweep the ground on the condition that I empty the trash cans).[17]

To introduce this transactional link between sponsors, researchers, and host communities, defenders of the economic model claim that "[t]he level of benefits that a community should receive to ensure a fair deal depends on the community's contribution relative to the contributions of all other parties that are involved in the research project, including sponsors, investigators, subjects, and other communities" (Gbadegesin and Wendler 2006, 251). Thus, we need to clarify if, and if yes, how a community could *contribute* to a research project within a *transaction* and in what sense communities hosting health research are prone to exploitation. Let us take a closer look at the alleged transaction between host communities and researchers with their sponsors.

Gbadegesin and Wendler (2006, 250) identify several criteria specifying when communities are actually *involved* and susceptible to exploitation in a transaction, that is, when research: "1) relies on the community's resources, including economic, social, knowledge based, or political resources; 2) focuses on the community's customs, traditions or practices; or 3) focuses on a health feature of the community." In the latter case, the argument is that individual members of a community could be exposed to the risk of stigma due to a certain health condition (e.g., HIV, in a community with high transmission rates); this stigma constitutes a burden (see Millum et al. 2019). Furthermore, the authors argue that whenever a community is involved in research according to one of these criteria, researchers and sponsors are likely to directly benefit from this involvement. It is the involvement of the community that allows the investigators and sponsors to conduct the study. Also, they benefit from the infrastructure without which a study would not be conductible. In short, Gbadegesin and Wendler's (2006) argument holds that community engagement establishes a special moral link between researchers/sponsors and communities. Fairness obligations arise from this moral link, and community exploitation is nothing other than failed compliance with these obligations.

However, this moral link—or "deontic link"[18] (O'Neill 1996)—is not obvious if we want to adhere to a *transaction-specific* account in order to explain community exploitation. As Wertheimer (2011, chap. 6) notes, the fair benefits approach can be criticized on the grounds that morally relevant transactions among investigators, sponsors, and host communities are not present. Unless the research places substantive burdens on communities, there is no obligation to share benefits fairly or to compensate for the burdens produced.[19] Moreover, and apart from these considerations, burdens to communities are mostly not greatly concerning. On the contrary, researchers and sponsors bring most of the resources expended to low-resource settings in less developed countries.

In research without substantive burdens for a community, Wertheimer (2011, 286–7) doubts that we can say that communities are exploited, or ground obligations of benefit-sharing toward host communities. Rephrasing Wertheimer's concerns, we face the following problem: international researchers and sponsors, A, take potentially exploitative advantage of the research subjects, B, but not of members of the host community, C (considered apart from those community members who are research subjects). The remaining question is whether A can exploit C in any way.

Hughes (2014) offers an account in which researchers and sponsors can exploit host communities either through their direct involvement in research (a direct transaction between A and C—a rarity) or through the mediation of exploitation by research subjects (the moral link between B and C is relevant to exploitation that occurs between A and B). Hughes (2014) does not see a moral genuine link that would explain the exploitation of communities by researchers and sponsors through a mutual transaction. The mere fact that researchers and sponsors interact with research subjects does not imply special, transaction-specific obligations[20] to broader communities. Thus, there are generally no special obligations of benefit-sharing toward host communities where one may suspect them (Hughes 2014). In consequence, there is no foundation for community exploitation. Nevertheless, even though researchers and sponsors do not have obligations in virtue of the way they interact with the broader host community, there are some special cases to consider.

Scenario 1: High Net Risk Research. In *high net risk* research, research subjects take risks not solely due to self-interest, but also for altruistic reasons. Thus, researchers and sponsors appeal to the broader perspective of a subject's altruism to serve a community. It would then not fair to ask citizens of impoverished host countries to take altruistically motivated risks if only high-income countries benefit (Hughes 2014). In this case, there may be special obligations on researchers to benefit host communities. Nonetheless, this argument has a considerable limitation: it would be perfectly reasonable to altruistically benefit *any* impoverished community or country around the world. There is no special obligation to benefit the host community in which a particular research study is conducted. Surely, one can criticize the non-relational account that Hughes (2014) defends here. Altruistic motivations on the part of research subjects could be tied to moral sentiments toward their fellow citizens.

Apart from that, there are greater problems at stake. First of all, assuming the altruistic sentiments of research subjects, at a general level, is epistemically weak. Research subjects may have nonaltruistic interests in accessing care facilities through clinical trials. Furthermore, Wertheimer (2011, Chapter 6) dismisses the idea that impoverished populations are "used" when research subjects are drawn from these populations. His point is that obligations toward communities are a *non sequitur*, meaning that they do not follow from the premise that research subjects are drawn from a community, as researchers and sponsors do not genuinely interact with or "use" the community in the way the "use" research subjects:

> (1) researchers use impoverished subjects drawn from an impoverished population; (2) researchers use the *improvised population* from which the subjects are drawn. But what does (2) mean? Certainly, the mere fact that research subjects are *from* a nation or community (1) does not mean that the researchers interact *with* or use a population in a way that could generate obligations to the community. (Wertheimer 2011, 285, emphasis present in the original text)

So, Wertheimer argues on the basis of a transaction-specific theory of exploitation that obligations toward communities cannot be grounded. The only situation that could give rise to obligations concerns direct burdens or adverse effects on communities. This means a direct interaction between A, researchers and sponsors, and C, communities, needs to be established.

Scenario 2: Public Resources. First, researchers and sponsors can place burdens on a community's resources; second, they can rely on the host community's public goods, such as infrastructure and public safety. In the first case, Hughes (2014) claims that researchers and sponsoring agencies should provide *fair compensation*. If they lay burdens on public resources without compensating an economically impoverished community, it would be unethical to conduct the research in this community. The same argument applies to a second case in which researchers and sponsors use the public goods of a community. Here, researchers and sponsors could commit the wrong of "free-riding." However, as long as researchers and sponsors actively contribute to the maintenance of the public goods they use in the course of research, they are not required to make special efforts beyond the provision of fair compensation.

Importantly, even though Hughes (2014) does not precisely tell us what fair compensation would entail, it is clear that it is some sort of monetary compensation for the use of public goods and resources, which does not necessarily concern the distribution of the net benefits generated through a research project. Fair compensation only requires that researchers and sponsors assure that communities are not made worse-off compared to the situation prior to the initiation of the research project. Differently put, it only demands that a community is not encumbered with a net burden. Thus, Hughes most likely considers fair benefit-sharing to be an obligation beyond the fair compensation of costs and burdens. Fair benefit-sharing concerns the distribution of the generated benefits in relation to the contributions of each party, and presupposes a concrete transaction.

Wertheimer addresses the problem differently. He argues that, first, it is not generally speaking true that an interaction between two individual parties A and B with harmful effects on other members of the community requires compensation:

> We sometimes think that the negative externalities of consensual and mutually advantageous transactions should lie where they fall. For example, if A hires B away from C (her previous employer), we do *not* generally think that A needs to compensate C. (Wertheimer 2011, 285)

Second, Wertheimer contends that research does not generally burden communities. If the research effort brings resources to the community that generate net benefits, it is hard to see why this would demand that researchers provide benefits to the community above and beyond what those already being provided. Here, Wertheimer makes his argument salient by referring to the example of movie companies, which, when filming on-location, often hire local "extras" and employ local hotels, restaurants, construction workers, and drivers (Wertheimer 2011, 286ff). Movie productions produce positive and negative externalities. On the one hand, rooms in hotels will be harder to find, traffic jams are more likely, etc. On the other hand, the movie company creates short-term employment and contributes to the local economy, which often outweighs the negative externalities. In this regard, the argument from burdening communities is not genuinely compelling.

Scenario 3: Direct Risks for Community Members. There are some forms of research that impose *direct* burdens or risks on individuals in host communities other than research participants. For example, in communities in which many people are genetically similar, publishing research results related to genetic features can have negative effects on community members, e.g., due to the risk of stigmatization of particular groups. However, as Hughes (2014) comments, even if we consider this kind of research compelling enough to establish that researchers and sponsors have a genuine special obligation to host communities, this type of research is infrequent in health research.

Following Wertheimer (2011, chap. 5) and Hughes (2012, 2014), we may come to the conclusion that the initial claim by Gbadegesin and Wendler (2006)—that communities have a claim on a fair part of the benefits produced through research—does not take us very far if we stick to the purely transactional paradigm. In particular, the normative architecture of the economic model is based on mutual and direct transactions between distinct parties. Fairness obligations can arise solely from individual transactions. As long as we do not explicitly show that host communities are directly exposed to unfair burdens and substantive risks in a transaction (or that they directly contribute to the generation of benefits), there are no transaction-specific obligations of fair benefit-sharing with host communities borne by researchers and sponsors. A groundwork for transactional models, and in particular a convincing framework for community exploitation, is still missing. At the end of the day, transactional models lack the justification requirement for fair benefit-sharing and the Exploitation Argument (Chapter 2) cannot be applied. The cases in which special obligations would emerge from an interaction, and the concept of transaction-specific exploitation would be applicable to a whole community, are very rare (Hughes 2014; Scenario 3).

Second Objection: No Account for Background Injustice

After having outlined a major conceptual problem associated with the ethical foundation of transactional models, we may nevertheless want to choose the transactional models under discussion and leave the problem of community exploitation aside. However, I will now present a second objection to transactional models that addresses a problem of so-called "background injustices." Background injustices find expression in unjust institutions, political and social injustices, and structural poverty (Malmqvist 2013). Poor countries that participate in international health research projects frequently lack developed legal systems or institutional structures, and do not adequately guarantee the redistribution of resources, basic goods, and/or basic liberties to their citizens.

To briefly sketch the common practice in international clinical trials, foreign researchers and sponsors are usually in contact with host institutions, such as local health authorities and ethics committees, to negotiate the terms and conditions of a research project. The problem of transactional models, and in particular the economic model, is that the focus on a hypothetically fair transaction between researchers and their sponsors and the local host community fails to acknowledge background injustices and the moral status of local institutions.

However, it is of great importance to know what kinds of institutions and agencies represent host communities. For instance, wouldn't it change the picture of a supposedly "fair" interaction if we knew that the government or the local health authorities were unjust institutions or even illegitimate representatives of their citizens? According to Mitra (2012) and Wenner (2015, 2018a), such problems gain importance in all cases in which benefits are disconnected from the social value of research designated to address local health needs. Such benefits all too often fall into the hands of corrupt institutions or accrue exclusively to the investigators and sponsors.

In the following, let's assume the justification requirement is met and researchers and sponsors have genuine obligations to share benefits with host communities. In other words, let's assume that communities can be established as stakeholders with legitimate claims toward researchers and sponsors.

The defenders of transactional models suggest that community members and research subjects are involved in a transaction via local institutions and community representatives; these function as guarantors of the community's interests and of a fair negotiation process (Emanuel and Participants 2008). There are at least two points related to background injustices that are completely ignored by transactional models, and most notably the economic model.

Community Exploitation and Background Injustice. My first point is connected to my more general objection to the economic model, which tries to ground community exploitation in a transaction-specific conceptualization of exploitation. But I do not mean to focus on the justification requirement. Here, I argue that we need to draw on a more comprehensive picture of how community exploitation is embedded in the broader context of justice and the fair distribution of benefits and burdens within a community.

Wertheimer's theory of transaction-specific exploitation ignores fundamental ethical issues on a macro-level. This leaves out a major worry: it is likely that local health authorities, contract research organizations, and representatives of the government do not represent the interest of communities, especially in LMIC contexts. It is possible that citizens of a LMIC country are exploited (assuming they can be exploited) because the local institutions do not adequately redistribute benefits.

The vulnerability model may be more cautious in this regard. In particular, the reasonable availability requirement demands that benefits from a research study must be made available on a large scale by implementing the tested medicines in a health care system or by selling the drug at lower prices. However, this is certainly not enough as a safeguard in contexts of significant background injustices. Consider for instance the scenario in which a country receives benefits, such as the provision of the tested intervention, which may be provided locally and covered by a local health insurance system. However, most of the country's citizens, and this includes especially impoverished and marginalized groups in low-resource settings (from which research subjects are often recruited), are not insured and thus, do not have access to the benefits of the intervention (Homedes and Ugalde's 2016). The point is: if we think that international researchers and sponsors gain from a host country and owe benefits in return (an assumption the economic and the vulnerability model sustain), we probably suppose that they owe those benefits not only to a subsection of cooperating individuals (most frequently, the rich or the insured) but to a fairly representative cross-section of the population. Thus, also the vulnerability model would need to address more seriously structural problems that potentially hamper the effective availability of medical interventions for a representative cross-section of the host population.

Here, my objection first and foremost addresses the missing acknowledgment of the link between the obligation of fair benefit-sharing (or the obligation to assure reasonable availability) and the structural working of systems. It returns to the initial objection I put forward against transactional models (Chapter 2). My argument is that transactional models isolate fairness considerations from the functioning of a cooperative system and fail to appropriately contextualize interactions between researchers, sponsors, research subjects, and communities as members.

Exploitation of Research Participants and Background Injustice. The second point concerns the direct negative effects of unjust background conditions on a very important subgroup of community members, namely, the research participants. There is a crucial moral point about the fact that international researchers and sponsors benefit and take advantage of background injustices to conduct ethically questionable clinical trials (Malmqvist 2013, 2017). According to many commentators, this is the case when researchers are not legally required to use an appropriate research design or to guarantee the post-trial provision of the tested intervention (London 2008; London and Zollman 2010; Malmquvist 2013, 2017). More specifically, in all these cases, unjust circumstances permit researchers and sponsors to conduct "cheap" research trials, such as trials under a double standard (Glantz et al. 1998; Macklin 2004a,b).

Wendler and Shah (2017, 7) argue that it seems unclear how background injustices could possibly pose an objection to transactional models. They claim that critics of the economic model, for instance, cannot convincingly show how the general obligations to address unjust background conditions in the world would be relevant to an ethical analysis of individual trials. There is one possible objection to this claim: background conditions influence even ideal (competitive) markets. This is the case when (random) background factors change the demand and supply to the detriment of one party. For instance, it is frequently argued that a lack of social institutions that normally adjust for misfortune and natural happenstance makes it more likely that the impoverished accept unfavorable terms of transaction in favor of more privileged agents who dominate them (see Vrousalis 2013). Arneson (2016, 16) puts the point this way: "the gains that people receive in a fully competitive market may not correspond to what they morally deserve or what they are entitled to according to sound principles of distributive justice." A price-taker cannot rule out the possibility that the terms she accepts are unfair in relation to her contribution and effort.

Likewise, one of the major problems concerning background injustices is that they impact on the transactions between researchers, sponsors, and research subjects.[21] Unjust background circumstances, such as a defective health system, make it more likely that individuals who participate in research accept unfair terms of transaction, as trials performed under a double standard show (see Malmqvist 2013, 2017, 2021). Structural injustices also frequently affect the functioning of local authorities that are or ought to be responsible for research oversight and the protection of research subjects (e.g., by guaranteeing that researchers and sponsors are complying with the terms agreed upon).

Third Objection: Unfair Distributions in Imperfect Markets

According to the logic of the economic model, fair benefits rely on "fair market allocations." The third problem I identify addresses the limitations of imperfect markets in attaining fair outcomes. The economic model wrongly presumes that negotiations happen on competitive and well-functioning markets in international health research.

It's worth mentioning that the fair benefits approach, or what I call the economic model, criticizes the vulnerability model on grounds of paternalism (Participants 2004, 21). The vulnerability model is paternalistic because it predefines the content of the benefits that should accrue to host communities. Defenders of the economic model argue that there is nothing in the model itself that requires host communities to accept only certain fruits of a particular research study when there are other benefits that those communities would like better (Participants 2004, 21). The economic model in fact allows for any sort of benefit that may result from research, including the ones outside the requirements of responsiveness and reasonable availability of the tested intervention. For instance, instead of offering a supply of a tested drug, researchers may help to establish a clean water supply or start a vaccination campaign in the host community (London and Zollman 2010). It strengthens communities' autonomy if they can decide on the terms of transaction they prefer (Emanuel 2008, 719–28, 724–5; see London and Zollman 2010).

Defenders of the economic model argue that the non-paternalistic approach aligns with uncoerced bargains between researchers with their sponsors and host communities in which the content of benefits is specified. This finds expression in a procedural account, which focuses on fair negotiation conditions from which fair outcomes automatically result.[22] Sponsors, researchers, and host communities are partners at the same table, engaging in a mutually advantageous bargaining procedure (Emanuel 2008; Emanuel and Participants 2008; London and Zollman 2010; Participants 2004). Transactional fairness under conditions of an ideal market plus compliance with fair procedural safeguards applied to the bargaining procedure yields outcomes that avoid exploitation (Participants 2004, 20).

However, London and Zollman (2010) have put forward a very valuable critique regarding the bargaining process. They criticize the economic model's third principle, namely, collaborative partnerships. Collaborative partnerships are the core mechanism the economic model offers to attain a fair distribution of benefits. The authors lament that collaborative partnerships do not offer specifics about how the bargaining process and the three criteria of fair benefit-sharing should be designed and implemented. For instance, one remaining question is whether bargaining is to be shaped in a way that makes it more likely to meet the condition of fair benefit-sharing or whether there is any additional oversight to assure a fair distribution of benefits. Here, London and Zollman (2010) come to the conclusion that the economic model is prone to unfair outcomes due to its "non-paternalistic" bargaining design. As long as LMIC communities agree upon a certain division of benefits, non-paternalistic bargaining may not genuinely be unfair or morally worrying, given that the host community freely accepts the bargain. However, if a free bargaining process leads to an unfair distribution, the result will contradict the aims of fair benefit-sharing.

London and Zollman (2010, 7) make the important point that the economic model and more precisely the mechanism of collaborative partnerships foster practices that allow sponsors to incur significant cost savings while being free to use their significant bargaining power to gain almost all benefits from the transaction. Therefore, they call the bargaining process an "auction" in which, at some point, communities will be willing to accept a level of benefits (surplus resulting from the study, minus costs) that is less of what it would cost another community to host the initiative. This is the case because international researchers and sponsors are in a monopoly-like position: they are able to negotiate freely with as many interested parties (host countries) as they like. Despite the transparent provision of sufficient information regarding costs, risks, and potential benefits associated with a particular research study, communities will eventually leave the negotiations without achieving the expected aim of a fair market price, as the lowest bidder wins.

Distorted markets are the main driving factor by which potential host communities bid for hosting the research (London and Zollman 2010, 8–19). Due to imperfect markets and a substantive lack of research oversight, the non-paternalistic aspiration of fair benefit-sharing does not work out in practice. This is the case even when transparent information about data regarding past bargains or better bargains would be available, as long as communities are not sufficiently empowered to negotiate on equal terms.[23]

To make it clear, this argument does not mean that LMIC communities do not have access to full or adequate information about the market. Indeed, the economic model suggests valuable mechanisms for making market information accessible to LMICs, e.g., through databases that historically trace back average benefits to other LMICs in similar negotiations (Emanuel 2008). The point here is, again, that communities cannot take advantage of these databases in "imperfect markets" resembling "auctions" to achieve better bargaining outcomes. Thus, solely procedural safeguards for fair bargaining defended by the economic model cannot prevent market distortions from converting research into an "auction block" with morally unjustified reservation prices.

Concluding Remarks

In the present chapter, I reconstructed and presented two common transactional models for the fair treatment of host communities in international health research, i.e., the vulnerability and the economic model, the latter also widely known as the fair benefits approach. My reconstruction results from an analysis of the debates on fair benefit-sharing starting in the 1990s. The models are reconstructed as transactional approaches because fairness obligations are not grounded in cooperative schemes across joint enterprises and agent networks but within transactions or negotiations between sponsors/researchers and representatives of host communities.

I presented three fundamental objections to the two transactional models. Perhaps my main achievement in this chapter has been to show that neither of the two models can fill the conceptual gap in the literature identified in the past chapter—that is, neither offer a valuable account of community exploitation or justify fair benefit-sharing with host communities in any manner (justification requirement). The postulation of obligations to the vulnerable and to transacting partners is no satisfying groundwork for fair benefit-sharing.

Furthermore, I introduced two practical objections to the current conditions under which offshored research is usually conducted. I argued that transactional models are unsuited to address the problems that arise from structural injustice, i.e., that benefits do not reach all community members and that the conduct of clinical trials under a double standard becomes more likely. Moreover, I demonstrated that the economic model, under its current design, is unlikely to safeguard fair benefits (or a fair share of the benefits at stake) due to distorted markets on which international clinical trials are "sold" to host communities. This objection is related to the content requirement of fair benefits.

This chapter clears space for the discussions in the following chapters, in which I attempt to find an alternative to the two transactional models at various different discussion levels. These discussion levels include the foundation of fairness obligations and community exploitation, the conceptual connection between transactional and structural injustice, and the content of fair benefits (including principles, procedures, and safeguarding mechanisms for fair benefit-sharing).

Part Three

Fair Play

4

Fair Benefit-Sharing and Community Exploitation under the Fair Play Model: Reply to Fundamental Objection (i)

From Transactions to Interactions

This chapter is concerned with the reconceptualization and normative grounding of the concepts of fair benefit-sharing and "community exploitation" in international health research. I here provide the groundwork that will later allow me to spell out the content of fairness obligations that transnationally operating sponsoring agencies and researchers bear toward host communities. As we have seen in the previous chapters, a brief genealogy of *fair benefit-sharing* and *community exploitation* suggests that our moral dissatisfaction in international health research concerns research enterprises that seem to exploit people in low-resource settings to the benefit of agents from the affluent world. I believe that the best approach to addressing the foundation of ethical obligations to host communities follows this historical debate. In plain terms, my strategy will be to argue that obligations of fairness arise as demands of nonexploitation and, vice versa, that the fair treatment of host communities—fair benefit-sharing—constitutes a condition in which communities are not exploited.[1] I consider this approach to be a defense and at the same time a valuable interpretation of the concepts so far introduced; it stands to reason and follows the research ethics tradition that started in the late 1980s and early 1990s.

My previous conclusion from Chapter 3 was that the conventional transaction-specific theory is too narrowly conceptualized to account for fair benefits and community exploitation. In my view, the focus on transaction-specific fairness has unjustifiably described the realm of "inter-actions" of researchers with their sponsors and communities. Interactions (from Latin *inter: between, amid* and *action: act of doing or making*) may involve more than single transactions (from Latin *transactio*: *completion, agreement, deal*); they may consist of multiple individual transactions either between individual agents or individuals and institutions that sometimes more or less linearly and sometimes only indirectly (in the background), e.g., trough tax payments, contribute to a common end. I use the term "interaction" relative to *cooperative schemes*, in which community members contribute to research without necessarily being counted as parties to duly arranged and fulfilled agreements between transacting partners.

G. A. Cohen's (2009) example of a camping trip in *Why Not Socialism?* intuitively explains what we might mean by cooperatively inter-acting (and not trans-acting) individuals: on a camping trip, resources brought along by people are shared, and people contribute variously to the necessary work according to their preferences and abilities. Some may cook, others wash up, still others fish, and so forth. The general idea is that everyone contributes in a public-minded way to a common end (Geras 2013, 235).

In this chapter, I will outline an account that can ground obligations that emerge in cooperative schemes, arguing that this is a reasonable theoretical foundation for fair benefit-sharing and community exploitation. I hope to offer a strong alternative to the transactional models discussed in the last chapter. In Section "Toward a Normative Model for Fair Benefit-Sharing," I argue that community members are legitimate stakeholders in research. Communities participate in a shared cooperative scheme under mutual restriction with the joint end of producing socially valuable knowledge together with researchers, sponsors, research subjects, local health agencies, and other stakeholders. This gives rise to obligations of fair benefit-sharing under Robert A. Phillips' (1997) stakeholder-specific adaptation of the principle of fairness, also known as the principle of fair play. I will call this approach the *fair play model*. Section "The Fair Play Model" fleshes out the concept of community exploitation under the fair play model, defined as the moral wrong researchers and sponsors commit when they do not comply with the principle of fairness. Then, I argue, they free-ride on the collective efforts of communities that help produce socially valuable knowledge in the course of a research enterprise. In Section "Objections to the Fair Play Model and Replies," I will defend the fair play model against four possible objections.

Toward a Normative Model for Fair Benefit-Sharing

A sound normative model to ground fairness obligations must, first of all, give defensible criteria for deciding which groups and individuals are and which are not stakeholders (answering the problem of appropriate stakeholder identity by explaining why a particular person or group is involved in a normative scheme while others are not). Second, it must suggest a principle by which different fairness claims of stakeholders are adjudicated; that is, it must regulate the distribution of benefits and burdens among the appropriate stakeholders. To avoid an important objection against the transactional model, such a principle needs to be of *political* scope, meaning that fairness obligations among stakeholders that arise under the principle must apply across *cooperative schemes.* I furthermore understand cooperative schemes as *relational entities* that consist of manifold members and manifold (including background) transactions in which members are involved.

Stakeholder theory after R. Edward Freeman suggests that there is a multiplicity of groups that have a stake in the economic operation of a corporation—all of whom are owed merit considerations (Phillips 1997, 52–3). Freeman (2010; Freeman et al. 2010) defines a stakeholder as any group or individual who can affect or is affected by the achievements of the corporation's objectives. As Phillips (1997) rightly notices, this is too broad and would include too many potential parties. Rather, it makes sense to presume that the basis for a group's engagement consists in the acceptance of the benefits of a cooperative scheme that creates an additional obligation owed to such groups. To identify a group as a stakeholder is to mark that group as meriting special consideration due to the presence of additional obligations (Phillips 1997, 54). This discussion relies on the foundation of (perfect) special obligations that are owed to a specified body of individuals and that do not arise from universal duties owed to everyone (O'Neill 1996, 152).[2]

But how do special obligations arise from engagement in a *collaborative scheme*? Strictly speaking, we do not only want to show that communities, researchers, sponsors, and other relevant stakeholders partake in research but that each of the contributors incurs an obligation to the other to perform her part. Differently put, we want to show that contributors acquire a claim-right to the others' performance and to a fair share of the benefits. There is a common possible account of how collaborative schemes can give rise to obligations, as follows.

Joint Agency

A common position held in the literature is that obligations may arise as a direct consequence of *joint agency*. According to Gilbert (1999, 2006), the presence of "shared intentions" or a "joint commitment" necessarily generates interpersonal obligations in collaborative schemes. Parties become creators of a joint enterprise through their personal commitment and owe each other conformity to the commitment. "In writing that members jointly accept a requirement of the form: members of P are to do A in C," Gilbert explains, "I mean to capture the idea that such joint acceptance amounts to the imposition of a requirement" (Gilbert 2006, 198).

Participating in a joint commitment means, by definition, to *accept* as a body some requirement that does not necessarily involve one's personal stance as an issue. But this does not mean any given individual personally requires that we all ought to do A in C (Gilbert 1999, 2006). Group rules are themselves grounding rights that commit each to conformity and corresponding entitlements, as well as impose pressure on noncompliant individuals. However, there is a substantial problem with the account itself. Many commentators think that obligations are not, at least, necessarily created through joint commitments. Gilbert's idea that all groups, *inter alia*, act as groups with a normative unity, a unity that gives rise to interpersonal obligations, is mistaken (Alonso 2008; Bratman 2014; Brigido 2010; Kutz 2000). To bring about normative unity, we need to show that the collective goal is sufficiently normatively valuable and just to create obligations, and/or that the group performing the joint action belongs to some normative scheme (Brigido 2010, 92).

The problem with Gilbert's (1999, 2006) account is that she considers a joint commitment to be obligation-creating, *per se* (Alonso 2008, 41f). To be binding, agreements or normative principles, like keeping promises, usually find expression in obligations and rely on just ends that are grounded in a commitment to a collective endeavor. If members are jointly committed then they are under an obligation to act accordingly *qua* members of the group. The nature of such an obligation is *conventional* in the sense that it is created by the "jointness" of a commitment (Alonso 2008, 68). However, there are examples of group members who are jointly committed, but do not bear obligations to comply with the group's collective goal, because the collaborative scheme is unjust. For instance, even though members of the *Camorra* might be jointly committed to certain ends, it does not follow that a single member would have any moral obligations to foster and comply with the syndicate's deeds and code of conduct. Jointness itself does not create obligations.[3]

The Principle of Stakeholder Fairness

I will proceed with an alternative approach to ground special obligations to host communities in large-scale collaborative schemes. Phillips' (1997) grounding of stakeholder theory in economic interactions is such an attempt. Phillips thinks that a principle of fairness or stakeholder fairness is ultimately needed to identify individuals or groups as stakeholders on the one hand (stakeholder identification), and to regulate the distribution of benefits and burdens on the other (distributive condition).

To clarify: using a theory of stakeholder fairness does not imply that there are no other, more intimate, and even stronger associative moral obligations (arising from other cooperative schemes) or universal duties (general obligations) beyond stakeholder fairness applying to members of a specified cooperative scheme. For instance, there may be obligations of egalitarian reciprocity among all fellow citizens *qua* members of a shared basic structure[4] (Sangiovani 2007; Wenner 2018a; see Rawls 1971, 1999a). A physician being involved in a research project may assume (voluntary) special obligations of fair cooperation to the sponsor and other stakeholders in the course of hosting a research project, and may have other (nonvoluntary) special obligations to the institutions of her country and her fellow citizens.

***

H.L.A. Hart is most often credited with the first explicit contemporary discussion of the "principle of fairness" or "fair play"[5] as a way to ground special obligations in collaborative schemes (Simmons 1979b, 101f). The principle was later taken up by Rawls (TJ, TJR), and was also complemented, criticized, and/or reformulated up to the present by a number of authors (see Arneson 1982; John and Millum 2020; Klosko 1989, 1992, 2005; Nozick 1974; Simmons 1979a,b, 2001; Spector 2014; Tosi 2018, and others).[6] In his essay "Are There Any Natural Rights?" Hart (1955) calls attention to a situation that he calls "mutual restriction" or "mutuality." He claims that there is an important source of obligations in a cooperative scheme that goes beyond the scope of what is mutually beneficial in transactions. According to Hart, the rights of the individuals who follow the rules in a cooperative scheme entail a corresponding obligation on the part of the beneficiaries. It is important to mention that the principle of fairness in Hart's version applies to individuals and the creation and maintenance of pre-institutional collaborative schemes[7] that are not necessarily identical with full-blown basic structures (Hart 1955, 185).

Hart's ideas have been well received by moral philosophers and contemporary political theorists. Most notably, John Rawls developed a version of "voluntary" fair play in a series of articles in the 1950s and 1960s in which he made various modifications to Hart's ideas:

> The principle of fair play may be defined as follows. Suppose there is a mutually beneficial and just scheme of social cooperation, and that the advantages it yields can only be obtained if everyone, or nearly everyone, cooperates. Suppose further that cooperation requires a certain sacrifice from each person, or at least involves a certain restriction of his liberty. Suppose finally that the benefits produced by cooperation are, up to a certain point, free: that is, the scheme of cooperation is unstable in the sense that if any one person knows that all (or nearly all) of the others will continue to do their part, he will still be able to share a gain from the scheme even if he

> does not do his part. Under these conditions a person who has accepted the benefits of the scheme is bound by a duty of fair play to do his part and not to take advantage of the free benefits by not cooperating. (Rawls 1964, 9–10)

Regarding the Rawlsian version of the principle, it states more explicitly (compared to Hart's account) the following points: First, there must be an active scheme of joint cooperation that is mutually beneficial and *just*. Second, benefits are potentially received by individuals that do not cooperate in return. In other words, there are potential free-riders who profit from the cooperative scheme (Rawls 1958; see Spector 2014; Simmons 1979a, 310f). Rawls later introduced the principle of fair play in *A Theory of Justice* (TJ, 108f) with the basic idea that no one ought to gain from the cooperative work of others without reciprocating a fair contribution.

The principle of fairness or fair play has furthermore been discussed in relation to the question of whether citizens have obligations to obey the laws of their countries, i.e., political obligations (Dagger and Lefkowitz 2014; Hart 1955; Rawls 1964, 117). Here, the principle of fairness serves as a foundational basis for the institutionalization of political obligations in societal structures and jurisprudence. Others have argued (or denied) that the principle of fairness or an adaptation of it is genuinely applicable to cooperative enterprises in which unrefusable public benefits, such as benefits resulting from the provision of public goods, accrue to a group of individuals and where some of those individuals potentially free-ride (Arneson 1982; Klosko 2005; Simmons 2001).

However, as I mentioned, I will follow a different theoretical adaptation of the principle of fairness, which has so far been used to conceptually underpin stakeholder theory in commercial interactions, a field that resembles to a great extent the particular case of health research. Phillips (1997) formulates the principle of stakeholder fairness as distinct from the original principle of fairness as it is known and discussed in the literature, precisely with the aim to adapt it to commercial interactions:

> *Principle of stakeholder fairness.* Whenever persons or groups of persons voluntarily accept the benefits of a mutually beneficial [and just] scheme of cooperation requiring sacrifice or contribution on the parts of the participants and there exists the possibility of free-riding, obligations of

fairness are created among the participants in the cooperative scheme in proportion to the benefits accepted. (Phillips 1997, 57, edited)

Phillips' fairness principle constitutes the basis for the following specifications (Phillips 1997, 57f). First, to create fairness obligations, an interaction between several stakeholders needs to create a mutual benefit or at least should aim to create a cooperative enterprise to the benefit of all stakeholders. Second, I add to Phillips' principle the requirement that the enterprise ought to be *relatively just*. This includes a just end and also a fair distribution of benefits and burdens (Klosko 1992, 39). Furthermore, it should be added that the "just end" condition presupposes that a collaborative scheme must pass independent moral tests.[8]

Third, Phillips (1997) specifies that benefits accrue despite conditions of near unanimity of cooperation. By unanimity of cooperation Phillips refers to the degree of joint commitment of cooperators to achieve a shared goal or to take advantage of a cooperative scheme. Phillips discards the unanimity condition, arguing that if all the other necessary conditions for fair play hold, it would be unfair to take the benefits of a cooperative scheme without contribution even if the benefits were obtained under conditions of substantially less than unanimity of cooperation (Phillips 1997, 55). This is important because when the possibility of large cooperative endeavors and many free-riders exists, obligations of fairness hold even if beneficiaries of the scheme are not committed to near unanimity.

However, collaborative schemes can be overinclusive if we completely discard the unanimity condition. The reason for that is that benefits in the form of positive externalities are multitudinous, often hardly calculable, and fall upon many (potentially unidentifiable) parties (Chauvier 2013, 70). Thus, I would like to contextualize what the condition of unanimity of cooperation may ask from cooperative agents. It might be right to say that we may suspect that every stakeholder is equally committed by near unanimity; however, there may still be an underlying, weaker *participatory interest* in a collaborative scheme. The intuition behind this is that both cooperation and the acceptance of benefits can proceed with a minimum of unanimity. Regarding the latter, the acceptance of benefits, an individual must be more than just a mere recipient of benefits or someone who happens to be affected by externalities.[9] Rather, she must willingly accept the fruits of cooperation (Simmons 1979b, 108). With respect to cooperation, already cooperating individuals can be ascribed a *participatory intention*, i.e., an individual role or performed act undertaken in order to foster a collective end. Here, the collective end is constituted by or is a causal product of different individual acts (Kutz 2000, 81). Using the example of an orchestra, Kutz (2000, 99) shows what participatory intentions are:

> [Suppose] a cellist plans to attend rehearsals, practice the cello part, attend the conductor's signals, and so on. But the cellist need not, and likely will not, engage in planning directed at ensuring that others will accomplish their parts, or worry about whether the bassoonists have properly realized the mood of the conductor's interpretation. (Kutz 2000, 99)

Participants, in this case the musicians, can *intentionally* contribute to an interaction without *intending* that the goal will be realized (Kutz 2000, 100).[10] This means they can have intentions to contribute without having the shared intention to realize a joint performance; and without taking on responsibility for another's part. The orchestra example hints at another interesting point: individuals can vary in the influence they actually have over the direction taken by the collective in choice of ends and means (Kutz 2000, 68–9). While the conductor takes the main direction and perhaps contributes significantly more to the success of playing the *Eroica* than a triangle player, we would still say that the trianglist has sufficiently overlapping participatory intentions to do her part in relation to the collective end.

Fourth, cooperation requires sacrifice or restriction of liberty on the part of participants in a collaborative scheme. According to Phillips (1997, 56), a commercial interaction underlies the principle of fairness most notably because all relevant stakeholders restrict their liberty in some significant sense. The most obvious case is that of an employee, who must sacrifice time and obey the rules of a company. The same happens with the exchange of property rights, e.g., when a community allows a company to build a plant on its territory, which implies a restriction on the liberty of the community to make different use of the territory, and also on the company that sacrifices some of its capital assets (Phillips 1997, 56).

Fifth, the possibility of free-riders exists. Free-rider conduct in cooperative enterprises with benefits to the members of a group emerges when individuals reason that all other persons contribute sufficient amounts to assure the continued operation of the scheme, even if they do not contribute to the costs or return adequate benefits (Arneson 1982; Phillips 1997). In this case, individuals are strategically better off not contributing and free-riding occurs. The principle of fairness is thus a moral constraint on free-riding that furthermore justifies penalties that can be enforced upon free-riders, assuring fair cooperation among individuals and the fair division of benefits and costs. This is at the heart of the principle of fairness, as suggested by Arneson (1982), Klosko (1992, 2005), Rawls (1958, 1964, 1971, 1999a), and Simmons (1979a,b).[11]

The free-rider problem is usually discussed as a case of market failure that occurs when those who benefit from a nonexcludable public good, such as a public resource or a communal service, do not pay for it, which in the long run leads to an under-production or degradation of the good (Arneson 1982; Cullity 1995). Free-rider conduct emerges in cooperative enterprises with *collective benefits* to the members of a group, given that the benefits for each individual are greater than the cost to her of contributing a fair share of the costs (including the costs of coercion to sustain the scheme) (Arneson 1982).

However, Phillips' "non-free-rider condition" should be understood differently (as not necessarily related to the benefits resulting from *public* goods). Stakeholders are suffering from free-riding in a commercial transaction "if [those] powerless stakeholders are unable to receive the full value of their sacrifices and contributions whether due to power differentials created by the organization [a firm], socioeconomic factors, or state power" (Van Buren 2001, 492). Free-riding here needs to be understood in a more general sense, as the failure to comply with a fairness norm, that is, failing to pay in proportion to the benefits received. Mayer (2007) captures this in the following way:

> Free riding offends what has come to be known as the principle of fair play, which requires individuals to reciprocate others' sacrifices from which they benefit. Beneficiaries must pay what others pay to produce the good, or pay in proportion to the benefits they receive, in order to avoid gaining at the expense of others. (Mayer 2007, 144)

This conceptualization of free-riding is, in the most general sense, related to benefits produced by a party A that accrue to another party B, where B fails to reciprocate benefits to A, or to bear a fair share of the costs. Feinberg (1990, 209) calls this "parasitism." In cases of harmful parasitism, we face a situation in which B behaves parasitically with respect to A, as B gains something that would otherwise go to A, so that his gain is A's loss. In cases of harmless parasitism (i.e., the "conventional" case of free-riding in the public good literature), B receives benefits from A's efforts without generating a loss in benefits for A. However, B fails to reciprocate the burdens necessary to generate these benefits.[12]

Last, the voluntary acceptance of benefits in cooperative (just and mutually beneficial) schemes creates fairness obligations. Originally, this condition was added by Rawls (TJ) and taken as a necessary precondition by other discussants of fair play, such as Nozick (1974), who claimed that voluntary acceptance should be tantamount to express consent. Following Phillips (1997), I will take it as axiomatic that consent is obligation-creating. At the core of the discussion, benefits obligate if they are accepted even by "tacit" or "implicit" consent (see Rawls TJ, 113). Phillips (1997, 59) makes that explicit by mentioning the example of a cooperative scheme among neighbors to provide an orchard:

> *The orchard example.* Suppose a neighborhood agrees that they all enjoy apples and wish to plant an apple orchard for the enjoyment of all. Such an orchard requires not only some rather hard work to get going, but also some maintenance throughout the year in order to yield the greatest number of high quality apples. Some neighbors explicitly consent and join the enterprise, while others do not. However, whenever a neighbor who has not consented eats apples from the orchard, she tacitly assumes obligations to return a fair contribution because the person actively and willingly partakes in the scheme of benefits. (Phillips 1997, 59, reconstructed argument)

Importantly, in this example, any agent can potentially opt out of the benefits. But the example also suggests that the acceptance of benefits immediately *creates* fairness obligations even if the relevant individual does not initially participate as a cooperator in the scheme. Thus, express consent adds nothing to obligations that already exist because *fairness* requires them.

Likewise, one can hold that by accepting benefits willingly, an agent expresses a participatory interest in the fruits of a collaborative enterprise and the *weak unanimity* condition is fulfilled.

Eventually, taken all together, economic interactions can be considered to give rise to cooperative schemes and stakeholders can be identified as all those agents who express a participatory interest, that is, participate as collaborators or accept benefits in some relevant sense (Phillips 1997; Van Buren 2001). The basic idea is that all stakeholder persons or groups are, even though to *varying degrees*, involved in the same cooperative scheme and the success of each is intertwined with the success of all others. Stakeholders are considered to be cooperators for mutual advantage and the principle of fairness serves as a norm that can be reasonably accepted by all parties involved.

The Fair Play Model

Let us now turn to the context of fair benefit-sharing in international health research. I propose a new ethical model to ground obligations, calling it the fair play model. I will argue that health research should be perceived as a cooperative scheme for mutual benefit, i.e., for the production of socially valuable knowledge, among researchers, sponsoring agencies, community members, research subjects, and other stakeholders, from which obligations to contribute one's fair share arise. I will show that community members are cooperative stakeholders in health research, even though they may not be directly involved in immediate transactions with foreign researchers and sponsors.

Research as a Joint Enterprise

There are many scholars who conceptualize research as a collaborative enterprise. Mitra (2012) and Danielle Wenner (2015), for instance, express the view that host communities are collaborators in research. The social value requirement consists in generating a socially valuable epistemic output that benefits future patients through the strengthening of a host community's capability to meet its basic needs or distinctive health priorities. In the same spirit, creators of research ethics guidelines actually consider the ultimate purpose of research to be the social output and contribution to the overall health improvement of a society that allows researchers to conduct studies (see CIOMS-WHO 2016, guideline 1; Emanuel et al. 2000; London 2005, 2012; Wenner 2015).

There is furthermore much consensus in the literature that the socially valuable benefits of research (like medical progress more generally) ought to accrue to a representative cross-section of the communities[13] from which research subjects are recruited (CIOMS-WHO 2016, guideline 1; Emanuel et al. 2004; Wenner 2015). For instance, let's take a look at the Havrix trial (Hawkins and Emanuel 2008, chap. 1; see also Chapter 1). Here, we understand the generation of socially valuable knowledge as a specific type of information that provides evidence for the safety and efficacy of a hepatitis A vaccine. If this information is to have some instrumental value for a representative cross-section of the community, it needs to be accessible to and shared with local leaders, authorities, researchers (e.g., hospitals, the Thai state, public health authorities, and local researchers), and reach out to potential patients. Moreover, the process of testing a vaccine creates valuable skills and knowledge for local health workers, which is useful for the conduct of future large-scale studies. These are all potentially value-creating activities that can arise from a research project.

If we define a research enterprise as a collaborative joint enterprise, we exclude demands that exceed the generation and redistribution of socially valuable knowledge *specific* to a given research project. External researchers and sponsoring agencies need not be committed (within the limits of the enterprise), e.g., to improve a country's general health system or infrastructure. These activities are outside the scope, the production, and sharing of socially valuable knowledge generated through research. Regarding the Havrix trial, this would exclude health services unrelated to the research project in which a hepatitis A vaccine is tested. However, this does not necessarily mean that researchers and sponsors are not allowed or should not be encouraged to perform such supererogatory activities. There may indeed be other duties of justice and beneficence beyond special obligations of fair benefit-sharing that ought to be discharged in the course of a research project (see discussion in Chapter 5).

Basic Structures—a Solution?

Danielle Wenner (2018b) offers the most successful foundational framework to account for "research as a joint enterprise" beyond the transactional models at present. Wenner (2018a) is one of the few scholars who have attempted to dig into the idea that research is a cooperative enterprise that is unlike transactions.[14] She suggests replacing the transactional model of research with what she calls a "basic structure model." The basic structure model is grounded in the claim that clinical research has a distinguished role in establishing the justice of our society and is thus subject to justice-based considerations like those in a Rawlsian basic structure, i.e., the design of the basic social and political institutions that structure daily life and individuals' decisions and actions, and which distribute fundamental rights and duties and determine the division of advantages of social cooperation (Freeman 2007, 464). Wenner frames this as follows:

> The correct model of the research enterprise is the basic structure model: Clinical research is one aspect of an institutional structure governing the health systems that are available to individuals, an institutional structure from which they cannot opt out, and which will have deep and lasting impacts on their life prospects, their final ends and purposes, and the way that they think of themselves. (Wenner 2018a, 31)

Thus Wenner (2018b) makes the epistemic output of research the target of justice-based principles regulating social cooperation. In her view, we can only justify research once we show that it is subject to a collective scheme in which all relevant stakeholders hold a valid claim to participate in the valuable outputs of such enterprise. The point here is that at the level of the basic structure of society, nobody can opt out; this means that every individual has a claim to participate in a scheme regulated by just institutions.

However, a basic structure is not the most fruitful theoretical foundation to capture the collaborative nature of international research projects (Holzer

2019). In my view, a cooperative enterprise does not necessarily presuppose a Rawlsian basic structure. This is due to the following reasons. A Rawlsian basic structure implies normatively relevant relationships among individuals who are subjected to a shared system of societal rules, institutions, and common law (Sangiovanni 2007). This concept thus falls under what is commonly known as a *strongly relational* account of justice and moreover, a *statist* account in which principles of justice apply specifically among people who, *qua* citizens of the same state, are required to act in accordance with just laws and institutional rules that regulate their lives. Here, the important idea is that people must stand *prima facie* in a certain relationship to one another to become subject to principles of justice. With the adoption of the basic structure model, Wenner (2018a) thus seems to follow a strongly relational account to characterize the type of collaborative enterprise present in health research. Although Wenner refrains from a univocal interpretation of "basic structure," she refers to a Rawlsian interpretation in which, she says, the social value requirement is founded in "major social institutions [that] distribute fundamental rights and duties and determine the division of advantages from social cooperation" (Rawls TJ, 7).

Now, the problem with a Rawlsian stance stems from the fact that in international health research, transnationally operating sponsoring agencies and sometimes investigators are external to the Rawlsian (domestic) basic structure of a host country. In the *Law of Peoples*, however, Rawls (LP, 33, 62, 114) outlines an international basic structure. Rawls asserts that peoples (or nations) are free and independent and should be respected by other peoples, that they ought to observe treaties and the mutually accepted rules of their "undertakings," and that they are equal parties to the agreements that bind them. This description, with its emphasis on mutual respect, resembles more the transactional model. To make a basic structure argument salient, one would need to show that sponsors, researchers, research participants, and community members together build a social scheme in which they participate *qua* members, subject to a shared system of societal rules, social cooperation, institutions, a common constitution, and law, as discussed by Rawls (TJ, TJR).

This claim may benefit from some empirical input. For instance, if a pharmaceutical company acts as a sponsor through a local branch or through locally operating contract research organizations (CROs) that are subject to the country's laws, we may argue that the sponsor is subject to a national social scheme by virtue of the local branch's participation in the domestic legal system (Stilz 2011). In this case, Wenner's (2018a) basic structure model indeed can make a very valuable normative contribution. However, this may not apply to the more general case I want to account for. There are many possible scenarios in which we do not consider sponsors and researchers to be members of a shared basic structure. Reconsider the Havrix Trial (Hawkins and Emanuel 2008; see also Chapter 1). The U.S. Walter Reed Army Institute of Research—embodying the US state—did not have the same membership (and thus moral) status as a local Thai sponsor would have had within a Rawlsian basic structure model. What's more: the US state is an institution pertinent to the basic structure, the political community of US citizens, representing the interests of US citizens and US companies, and being financed by US tax money.

Admittedly, more work needs to be done to evaluate whether the basic structure model could be salient to international health research.[15] For my purposes, I will solely pursue the strategy to establish community members as stakeholders within collaborative schemes together with international researchers and sponsors. Doing this has the advantage that I do not need to explain why cooperators belong to certain ethnic, cultural, political communities, or overarching global basic structures, while still accounting for the interest of community members to partake in the fruits of research.

The Fairness Principle Applied to International Health Research

I argue that Phillips' (1997) principle of fairness, when applied to the context of international health research, can offer a satisfactory account. The principle is able to establish community members as valid stakeholders within a cooperative scheme, without presupposing a basic structure, and grounds obligations to share benefits fairly among stakeholders. I will demonstrate that the requirements of stakeholder fairness outlined in Section "The Principle of Stakeholder Fairness" hold for the case of international health research.

Research Creates Mutual Benefit

First, a cooperative scheme needs to be designed as a scheme of *mutual benefit*. Ideally, the anticipated research outcome of clinical trials should be socially valuable knowledge, i.e., benefits in the form of health data that are potentially valuable to a representative cross-section of the participating stakeholders. To further show that international health research is a *benefit-creating* activity, Robert Levine (2008), one of the founding fathers of bioethics, argues that research produces an important good in the most general sense, from which mutual benefits can subsequently be derived (see Section "Research as a Joint Enterprise"):

> It [biomedical research] has as its purpose the advancement of goals that are greatly valued by our society—enhancing the capabilities of physicians (and other health-care professionals) to serve the health interests of people. Some biomedical research projects do this directly and others indirectly by adding to or refining the fund of knowledge that provides the basis for future therapeutic innovations and improvements. (Levine 2008, 215)

Here, Levine depicts biomedical research as an enterprise that aims to produce collective benefits because knowledge creation is directly instrumental to the goal of good health of our societies: it enhances the capabilities of health workers, provides improved medicines and technologies, and enriches a fund of knowledge that is necessary for future innovations and improvements.

Another founding father of research ethics, Hans Jonas (1969), argues that "health" is served directly by physicians and indirectly by the knowledge gained through experiments. However, research has first and foremost a melioristic goal (Jonas 1969, 230). It does not serve the preservation of an existing good or state of welfare from which someone profits and to which people are obligated to contribute (Jonas 1969, 230).

From Jonas' viewpoint, research is beneficial, but not strictly essential in the sense that it is not directly important for a fulfilling life *if* life is not intolerable in the present state with the present standard of health and health care. The central good at stake remains *health*, not medical advancement. Our intuition may be, nevertheless, that research constitutes a somewhat "auxiliary" good, namely knowledge, which is nevertheless necessary not only to foster but also to maintain the good of health and health care, to respond to global health threats and challenges, and to alleviate suffering and cure diseases. Qualitative medical care always relies on medical innovation, improvement, and knowledge (see Holzer and Mastroleo 2018; London et al. 2010).

Thus, we may follow Levine in contending that the social value of research is an essential good for society, and not a mere melioristic good. To expand on Levine's claim, we ultimately owe part of our living standard, life expectancy, and health care standards to biomedical research, which justifies the expenditure of public resources and the exposure of research subjects to risks (Emanuel et al. 2000). Many diseases, such as tuberculosis, malaria, and other infectious diseases, affect the global poor and leave them destitute (Banerjee et al. 2010). The generation of socially valuable knowledge promotes public health, disease prevention, and treatments, which have already significantly reduced human suffering (Chen et al. 1999). Research thus contributes to the general well-being of people and has also a significant positive impact on broader social and political factors, such as work conditions, the economy, and education (Daniels 2008; Venkatapuram and Marmot 2009).

Nonetheless, there may be an important objection to the claim that health research produces an essential good with mutual benefits for a considerable cross-section of a society (or humanity), such as community members. More specifically, there may be research with "low social value," such as research on rare diseases that only serves very few individuals and does not produce large-scale benefits. I cannot say much in few lines, as the objection requires a more in-depth analysis of conceptions of socially valuable knowledge, rights of minorities and the worst-off, pluralism, fair participation, and democracy in science (see, e.g., Barsdorf and Millum 2017; Del Savio 2017; Kitcher 2011). I will not deepen this objection here and only reply briefly: according to Varmus and Satcher (1997), the burden of disease in developing countries is a valuable reason to make research studies ethically compelling. Studies that are outside the focus of a country's health needs would work against the general interest of communities, as they do not come along with sufficient collective benefits. They claim: "Might we elect not to support a trial of an intervention that was beyond the reach of the citizens of the other country? Yes, because that trial would not pass the test of justice" (Varmus and Satcher

1997, 1003–4). "[N]ot passing the test of justice" means that research lacks a just end, i.e., a sufficient *mutual* benefit for all cooperating parties involved and lacking an end that does not violate *prima facie* our most basic moral intuitions (Dworkin 2011). Hence, mutual benefit and sufficient social value seem *prima facie* necessary when applying the principle of fairness to international health research.

The Justice Condition: Just End and Fair Cooperation

The justice condition of the principle of stakeholder fairness entails two dimensions: a just end and a fair mode of cooperation. Regarding the first dimension, research is plausibly an enterprise aimed at producing an essential good, namely socially valuable knowledge; it thus yields potential health benefits to all. Maintaining and enhancing health means serving an essential interest and a just end shared among people. According to Daniels (2008, 145), health can be regarded as essential to an individual's normal functioning, which in turn is a necessary condition of pursuing one's individual life plans. However, this does not automatically imply the second dimension of justice, i.e., that the collaborative scheme is just. The principle of fairness generally regulates cooperative enterprises where benefits produced by cooperators accrue to others. I especially consider the justice condition as a demand that every stakeholder ought to discharge the fair contribution that corresponds to her in relation to the reception of benefits from cooperation. The justice condition therefore morally binds an individual party to do her fair share and to support an *ex ante* just cooperative scheme. The general idea expressed by the principle is that it is wrong for people to be exempt from burdens others bear or to take a disproportionate share of the benefits at stake, as there are no morally relevant differences between equal parties.[16]

A joint enterprise must be presumably (and at least moderately) just in order to create obligations on participants in a collaborative scheme. This should be understood in the most general sense, meaning that I haven't said anything about how one ought to discharge these obligations. The principle of stakeholder fairness seems to be a promising candidate principle to justify obligations of fair benefit-sharing in international health research, as questions in this context turn around the fair distribution of cooperative benefits in a presumptively just enterprise where one party, however, potentially benefits more from the generated collective benefits without returning a fair share. I assume that the generation of socially valuable knowledge is presumptively just and benefit-creating, but international researchers and sponsors often benefit *disproportionally* more. This is supported by historical case studies in the literature, current examples from international health research, and the growing awareness of neglected community interests and calls for fair benefit-sharing in the literature since the 1990s (Glantz et al. 1998; Hawkins and Emanuel 2008).

The point here is that once we interpret health research as a collaborative scheme, we assume that the host community delivers a substantial contribution to the enterprise by providing the background environment for health research, including health staff, institutes, infrastructure, security, and the research subjects recruited from the communities. Wendler and Rid (2017, 83) explain that there are further, project-specific contributions. For example, the products researchers and sponsors test may have previously been tested in publicly funded laboratories; human resources, such as laboratory assistants, nurses, and other health workers are drawn from the local population. It is true that sponsoring agencies, investigators, and research subjects certainly make a project-specific contribution when they either provide themselves as test subjects, employ their expertise to conduct research, or finance the research and development process. Background and some project-specific contributions by community members are furthermore necessary to achieve the completion of both single projects and research understood more broadly. Community members, however, usually do not shape the revenue-generating properties of a particular project, such as the operational and organizational basis of a clinical trial (Wendler and Rid 2017, 83–4).

In terms of the orchestra analogy, it is true that the conductor and soloists contribute considerably and directly to the successful performance of the *Eroica* (Kutz's 2000, 99). So do sponsors and principal investigators with regard to a research project. Depending on the magnitude of their contributions, research subjects, research monitors, and nurses may be comparable to the musicians. But the eventual success of the *Eroica* does not only depend on the orchestra but on a variety of different offices and contributions in the background. These background contributions concern music as a cultural activity. For instance, a concert hall must be maintained, and tickets must be sold; someone must be in charge of the sound, the lights, etc. We may draw the analogy between these jobs and community members who fall under the category of background contributors. Importantly, not being the center of attention does not deprive them of their legitimate role as contributors to the collective end; they deserve proportionate remuneration.

Subsequently, researchers and sponsors are bound to the obligation to contribute and return their fair share to an enterprise in virtue of the benefits they receive from and thanks to communities. This implies more concretely that research needs to show *ex ante* a sufficient possibility of generating social value for communities because otherwise, there is no possibility that communities are afforded a fair share of the benefits. A fair share can foreseeably be returned only if a research question is significant enough to produce—for a community—valuable knowledge and if a community's health system is sufficiently *well functioning* to transform socially valuable knowledge into a health benefit for a considerable cross-section of the locals. Thus, when researchers and sponsors are morally bound to cooperate fairly in a joint enterprise, they must ensure that these preconditions exist. Apparently, researchers and sponsors as primary contributors to a joint project often create benefits that accrue to a host community. However, their average return and efforts to produce social value for communities (and this is the controversial point in the history of research ethics) may be not enough under a principle of fair play, as they are morally required to return a *fair* share, not merely *a* share.

Unanimity and Cooperation

As I previously explained, I contend that a weak form of unanimity needs to be present among cooperators for them to qualify as stakeholders. This does not mean cooperators must have the same (joint or group-) intention to contribute to and identify with a common end (Kutz 2000, 100). The parties may all have distinct interests that lead to their participation in a joint enterprise: researchers and sponsors have economic interests; research participants, individual interests to access medicines and ancillary care facilities; and community members, interests in receiving future health benefits.

Nevertheless, health research cannot be separated from its initial justification, which sets a collective goal, i.e., the creation of socially valuable knowledge to foster and maintain health and medical progress. Here, I shall distinguish between research as an activity and individual research projects. Research as an activity always aims to serve the fundamental interest of community members and, more generally, humanity (CIOMS-WHO 2016; Emanuel et al. 2004; Levine 2008; London 2005; Nuremberg Code 1949, principle 2; Snyder 2012; Wenner 2018a). A particular research project, even though a short-term activity, ought to be seen as an individual action to produce knowledge that (generally) aligns with the long-term collective goal of fostering health.

Thus, it is possible to claim that stakeholders contribute to the goal of producing socially valuable knowledge to foster health under the condition of (at least) weak unanimity. To sustain a notion of weak unanimity and some sort of collaborative scheme, it is necessary to show that every agent is recognized as having a particular causal role (and thus a *participatory* intention) in *fostering* this end (Kutz 2000, 104–5). While it seems more evident that researchers, sponsors, and research subjects are directly involved in contributing to the generation of knowledge, the orchestra analogy allows us to claim that communities also contribute in the background to this collective end. Transactions and activities in the background, such as the training of health workers, or the maintenance of health facilities, and most notably institutional interactions, like tax payments or the maintenance of national security, build together the structural basis for (and indispensable contributions to) research.

Mutual Restriction of Liberty

The previous characterization of communities as sufficiently unanimous cooperators for the achievement of mutual benefit eventually brings us to Phillips' (1997, 56) most pivotal requirement of stakeholder fairness, which is necessary to establish a party as a fully recognized stakeholder. An interaction gives rise to fairness obligations borne by a party A if a party B restricts her liberty in some significant sense so that party A is benefiting from that restriction and is thereby helped in achieving her goal. As in Phillips' general case of commercial interactions, community members in health research can be established as stakeholders due to their background contributions, which arguably consist of significant restrictions of their liberties to achieve the production of socially valuable knowledge. This restriction first and foremost concerns the payment of taxes to maintain research facilities, the education of health workers, and the maintenance of public goods necessary for a successful interaction; it may also concern additional health care services for research participants. It is important to note that research causes an increased burden, i.e., increased taxes, by otherwise stable tax payments for other social goods. Putting it the other way round, research implies investments that have opportunity costs; that is, other valuable alternatives are forgone in favor of the chosen option to foster research. Precisely because community members restrict their liberty in this relevant sense, and researchers and sponsors obtain benefits from this restriction, obligations of fairness arise in this mutual engagement, which means that community members have a claim to a comparable restriction on the part of researchers and sponsors (Hart 1955, 185; Phillips 1997, 56).

The Possibility of Free-riding

At the heart of the principle of (stakeholder) fairness is that fairness obligations serve as a restraint on free-riding (Arneson 1982; Klosko 1992, 2005; Phillips 1997; Rawls 1964; TJ, TJR; Simmons 1979a,b). As I said, free-riding has to be understood in a general sense, as what Feinberg (1990, 209) calls *parasitism*, where a party B receives benefits from A's efforts without reciprocating benefits or burdens necessary to generate these benefits (see Chauvier 2013, 199ff).

I argue that what Feinberg calls "parasitism" can occur in international health research (Feinberg 1990, 209). Researchers and sponsors frequently benefit from infrastructure, including public goods, such as security, clean water, and other public resources necessary for research, as well as educated workers and sanitary facilities. There is the risk that they do not fairly compensate communities for receiving those benefits. Researchers and sponsors then commit free-riding on pure public goods or on the uncompensated use of resources. Furthermore, researchers and sponsors often make use of, from their view, "favorable" circumstances, which make disease testing possible. Consider, for instance, the Trovan case (introduced in Chapter 3), in which Pfizer tested the drug Trovan in individuals with cerebro-spinal meningitis in Nigeria, where an outbreak of the disease occurred. According to Okonta (2014, 190), Pfizer "left the town after conducting the study despite the fact that the epidemic was still ongoing." It seems that Pfizer took advantage of an outbreak, the health conditions of research participants, and a developed infrastructure that allowed for the pursuit of drug testing without reciprocation or compensation of the community.

Nevertheless, in many instances, monetary contributions to infrastructure, public goods, and resources exist and fair compensation is fulfilled (see Hughes 2012, 2014). This was most likely the case in the Havrix trial, where enormous efforts were made to modernize the infrastructure and to train health workers (Hawkins and Emanuel 2008). However, when considering research as a collaborative enterprise, in which all stakeholders contribute to the generation of socially valuable knowledge, we imply a considerable restriction of every party's liberty and opportunity costs. Despite the fair compensation of public goods and resources, researchers and sponsors may still take unreciprocated advantage of the *general efforts* (including background contributions and opportunity costs) made by community members to generate knowledge, which, in turn, can be transformed into economic profit via patents that allow selling an approved drug under a monopoly price.[17]

Now, if it occurs that the return of the epistemic output from research solely or mostly accrues to researchers and sponsoring agencies and not to a community (and research participants), we face a form of parasitism *in relation to the production of knowledge*. This is the case when researchers and sponsors return insufficient benefits to a community given its contribution to the potential knowledge gain. More specifically, this occurs when there is an insufficient transformation of knowledge into health benefits related to a research activity, namely, the idea that socially valuable knowledge improves health systems that attend to patients' needs in the form of updated clinical care, improved treatments, updated knowledge, local capacities, and health services (Mitra 2012). In view of the significant contributions by communities, we may expect from research that community members should be able to draw benefits from knowledge attained through research and from improved public health systems as potential patients.

The fair benefits approach (Emanuel 2008; Emanuel et al. 2004) seems to offset this "insufficient gain" from the knowledge production by arguing that compensatory benefits can be provided to communities as to assure that communities obtain an ideally "fair" net benefit. Arguably, researchers and sponsors are the primary agents that create socially valuable knowledge alongside other valuable benefits, such as the creation of jobs at the research site, training of health personnel, or the modernization of infrastructure.

So, is a trade-off between those benefits justifiable? One may argue that training health personnel and improving infrastructure are required in order to conduct a clinical trial and produce generalizable knowledge. So, it may be problematic to count all these necessary costs as benefits for communities. However, even if costs borne by researchers and sponsors are considered at the same time benefits for communities, fairness under the principle of stakeholder fairness is understood to be relative to the benefits and burdens that occur in a collaborative scheme with the aim of producing knowledge. So, even if researchers and sponsors are providing communities with additional benefits unrelated to the research enterprise, those communities may still benefit less, proportionally, from the knowledge that results from the collaborative enterprise. Placing researchers and sponsors under the principle of stakeholder fairness in a collaborative scheme is therefore tantamount to the claim that researchers and sponsors are otherwise (potentially) free-riding on the efforts of a host community when drawing disproportionally high benefits from the generation of knowledge, given the burdens and costs communities bear.

Voluntariness

Phillips' (1997) fairness principle states that the benefits of a collaborative scheme must be voluntarily accepted in order to incur obligations. Accepting benefits does not presuppose express consent, as Phillips demonstrates in the orchard example. Now, it is true that a sponsoring agency together with researchers from abroad indeed voluntarily accept benefits. From their view, moreover, it may be obvious that once other stakeholders accept benefits from the research enterprise they initiate, fairness obligations are also placed upon these other stakeholders, such as host communities. But the "voluntary acceptance" in both cases is asymmetric (Van Buren 2001). For voluntary acceptance to be meaningful, some hypothetical consent must be freely given, informed, and not coerced, which means that highly unfair schemes can never truly be consented to. The "justice condition" would not allow for valid consent in such a context.

Moreover, non-ideal circumstances often lead to significant powerlessness, which means that the acceptance of benefits is not always done voluntarily and fairness obligations based on the acceptance of benefits cannot always be incurred. Van Buren's (2001, 490) central point is that where meaningful consent exists, fairness will also exist. For a research enterprise to be a truly cooperative scheme for mutual advantage of all stakeholders, consent (either explicit or hypothetical) and/or the acceptance of benefits must be taken up as a means of ensuring fairness. The principle of fairness thus takes up a crucial point about the issue of accepting benefits: the acceptance of benefits is already intrinsically connected to whether (roughly speaking) fairness in stakeholder relationships exists.

However, this concern is not fundamental to the grounding of fairness obligations that *researchers and sponsors* incur. In the revised edition of *A Theory of Justice*, Rawls (TJR) may offer us an explanation: principles of natural duty to comply with and support just institutions apply to all citizens and are derived from a contractarian point of view; this means that they do not presuppose an act of consent, express or tacit, or the voluntary acceptance of benefits. In turn, voluntarily incurred obligations arising from the principle of fairness usually establish bonds that support existing *just* arrangements. Here, and this is essential in Rawls, the principle of fairness (also in a pre-institutional context) primarily applies to the *better-situated*:

> The principle of fairness … binds only those who assume public office, say, or those who, being better situated, have advanced their aims within the system. There is, then, another sense of noblesse oblige: namely, that those who are more privileged are likely to acquire obligations tying them even more strongly to a just scheme. (Rawls TJR, 100)

Rawls' (TJR) principle of fairness serves to ensure that those who have the privilege to advance their interests have fairness obligations toward others who can perhaps not advance their interests in the same autonomous way. This insight is crucial not only for the context of a basic structure but also in the pre-institutional context of a cooperative scheme in health research: Van Buren's concern about whether community members who "voluntarily" accept the benefits of research are actually placed under fairness obligations is of secondary importance. If interpreted in the Rawlsian way, fairness obligations primarily fall on those who have the privilege to advance their interests voluntarily through a mutually beneficial cooperative scheme. Researchers and sponsors are better-situated parties in a research enterprise that takes place in a LMIC context against a background of non-ideal circumstances and against asymmetric power relations among relevant stakeholders. In this regard, it suffices to prove that these agents bear fairness obligations once they accept the benefits resulting from the restriction of other (frequently worse situated) stakeholders' liberties in a collaborative scheme.

Wrapping Up the Fair Play Model

After having shown how Phillips' (1997) interpretation of the principle of fairness can be specifically applied to the context of international health research, I would like to summarize the basic insights gained from the last sections and further develop the fair play model. At the heart of the fair play model is the claim that fairness obligations arise from cooperative schemes for mutual benefit. This allows us to draw a clearer distinction between stakeholders and non-stakeholders. Parties that are not concerned by Phillips' fairness principle, i.e., parties that do not sacrifice, contribute, or restrict their liberty in any significant way in relation to the end of a joint enterprise—and on a strict interpretation, do not voluntarily or willingly accept the benefits of a mutually beneficial scheme of cooperation—cannot be considered stakeholders. Phillips' theory of fairness has therefore both an identification component, which identifies stakeholders, and a normative component that names distributive justice as the ethical decision rule: fairness obligations are created among the participants in a cooperative scheme in rough proportion to the benefits received and the burdens borne (Van Buren 2001, 485).

I construct an argument in favor of the view that transnationally operating researchers, sponsors, host communities and other stakeholders build a collaborative scheme because they all jointly contribute to a collective end, either through positive background contributions or through direct contributions to an individual research project with the aim of producing socially valuable knowledge. This specific group constellation is pre-institutional and *not* specific to a basic structure, ethnicity or cultural community features, in which individual parties cannot opt out from participating, as researchers and sponsors may leave the joint enterprise after conducting a particular research project. Also, the collaborative enterprise is specific to a joint aim, i.e., the production of knowledge, which does not extend to other spheres of interaction among the participating parties. The primary justification of research is related to the production of knowledge, and not to potential positive "side benefits," such as, e.g., an improved infrastructure. "Fair benefits," as a fairness norm, are achieved when a sufficient (i.e., proportionally fair) amount of benefits resulting from the knowledge production is returned to communities. To convert knowledge into real (health) benefits, health systems and services must be sufficiently well developed, or measures must be taken to help communities in the conversion process.

The fair play model eventually answers the identification problem of stakeholders. It suggests that stakeholder identification succeeds based on cooperation, and not on a communitarian view; that is, the fact that research participants belong to a community does not automatically imply that community members hold special claim-rights. Only cooperators in the relevant sense, as specified by the fairness principle, are stakeholders and have a claim to fairly partake in the benefits created under cooperation. This claim-right is proportional to an individual party's contribution, her restriction of liberty, and presupposes that a cooperator has an individual role in a collaborative scheme, meaning that at least the weak unanimity requirement is fulfilled. Usually, weaker unanimity between cooperators goes along with fewer contributions. So, it may be true that community members at the research site, e.g., members of a municipality from which research subjects are recruited, show a higher degree of involvement: in some countries, the municipality takes care of the research facilities, educates and provides health workers, provides care for research participants, and frequently engages in a community-centered orientation-based dialogue, or what is commonly described as "community engagement."

However, research construed as a collaborative scheme is more inclusive: individuals in the wider context of a country also contribute positively in the background and thus restrict their liberty in a relevant sense for a joint end, most notably via tax payments for public goods and for project-specific research funding, or the maintenance of facilities;[18] and, generally speaking, by the opportunity costs they bear. They ideally benefit when the generation of knowledge adds to an improved health system, health care, or better policies. Here, the fair play model offers an account that can explain why more benefits are owed or should be granted to cooperators compared to non-cooperators with similar or worse health needs, e.g., communities in countries other than the host society.

The fair play model takes into account the different degrees of involvement, contributions, and fairness claims of distinct community members. Background contributors in a community (e.g., understood as the citizens of a host country)[19] certainly hold a weaker claim-right to benefits, perhaps not strictly comparable with the claim-rights of direct contributors, such as research subjects and members of the local community at a research site. However, the fact that increased tax money (or constant tax money accompanied by increased opportunity costs) and other concessions in the background are directly contributing to the successful realization of the joint end of producing socially valuable knowledge means that researchers and sponsors are not exempt from general fairness obligations toward citizens of host countries.

The fair play model exhibits considerable advantages compared to the ethical models so far presented in this book, that is, the basic structure and the two transactional models for fair benefit-sharing. On the one hand, research as a joint enterprise (collaborative scheme) does not run into the same problems as transactional models do when they try to establish community members as stakeholders. As I previously stated, a joint enterprise is an entity beyond transactions (see Alonso 2008, chap. 1). More precisely, a joint enterprise can consist of multiple transactions which all, directly or indirectly in the background, foster the joint end of a collaborative scheme. This allows us to account for community members as fully recognized stakeholders. Here, community members do not participate in a specified "transaction" with researchers and sponsors; they, however, participate in a joint enterprise, most of them as background contributors.

On the other hand, the most developed and promising contemporary alternative to the transactional account seems to be the basic structure model (Wenner 2018). The basic structure model does not struggle to integrate community members as legitimate stakeholders. The difficulty lies in the argument that external agents participate in a basic structure. Then, framing research as a joint, but pre-institutional, enterprise is a good middle way: while leaving behind the transactional modus in which communities, researchers, and sponsors cannot be tied together under the label "collaborative scheme," I do not need to commit myself to the postulation of strong normative relationships between those agents in a shared relational scheme like a basic structure.

Community Exploitation under the Fair Play Model

In Chapter 2, I anticipated reinterpreting fair benefit-sharing and community exploitation, thus providing a reformulated exploitation argument—which is necessary to yield a defensible justificatory groundwork for the fair treatment of host communities. Remember, the exploitation argument, previously advanced by Angell (1988), Varmus and Satcher (1997), Glantz et al. (1998), and Wenner (2015, 77), provides an intuitive justification for the requirement that research ought to produce socially valuable knowledge for communities: communities are exploited if they cannot derive a fair share of socially valuable benefits from the knowledge produced by research.

This reconstruction of the exploitation argument appeals to the question about distributive justice, i.e., fair benefit-sharing. Socially valuable knowledge produced in well-designed research must be "tailored" or sufficiently transformed into health benefits for a host community to avoid exploitation of communities in a collaborative scheme. My present account suggests rejecting the transactional model in favor of a fair play model that entails fairness obligations based on the interaction of relevant stakeholders in a collaborative scheme. Fair benefit-sharing means that stakeholders in research ought to comply with the obligations that apply to them under a certain fairness norm, which, I argue, ought to be the principle of stakeholder fairness. This captures what is at the heart of the exploitation argument: if researchers and sponsors do not comply with the obligation to cooperate fairly in a joint enterprise, which they acquire in virtue of the principle of (stakeholder) fairness, they exploit other parties.

Host communities are frequently among the exploited, that is, among the stakeholders that obtain too little of the benefits at stake. The exploitative nature of research lies in asking communities to contribute to a collaborative scheme from which they derive little or no benefit as potential patients (see Mitra 2012, 5). I will eventually interpret this as "community exploitation" in light of the above analysis. Theories of exploitation, including Wertheimer's (1999, 2011) transaction-specific theory, have all along contributed to a contentious debate in research ethics (see Malmqvist 2013, 2017; Mitra 2012; Snyder 2012). There have been some attempts to capture the specificities of community exploitation (see Glantz et al. 1998), but most theories in research ethics have established a conception of exploitation confined to transactions and the partial relationship between exploiters and exploited (Emanuel and Participants 2008; Participants 2004; Resnik 2003). The transaction-specific focus on exploitation, which is certainly of great importance to most types of exploitative scenarios, has confused the conceptualization of community exploitation, a confusion that most notably comes into effect in the transactional economic model (Emanuel 2008; Participants 2004).

Rather than enumerating the components of a defensible concept of exploitation, I argue that community exploitation in the fair play model is equivalent to free-riding (or what Feinberg [1990] reframes as parasitism) on the efforts of community members who collaborate in the production of socially valuable knowledge within a joint enterprise. The moral wrong of free-riding can offer us a valuable and moreover intuitive explanation of why the exploitation argument is important. As I previously stated, Mayer (2007, 138) introduces the concept of "free-rider exploitation" as the failure to benefit another party as fairness requires. Community exploitation is, by my definition, the opposite of fair cooperation, or, put differently, noncompliance with fairness obligations as the principle of fairness requires it.

Finally, I would like to bring forward two more clarifying points. First, my interpretation of community exploitation remains narrow in the sense that it does not rely on other factors, e.g., the *status quo* of background injustices (remember, I criticized the transactional models for being insensitive to background injustices in Chapter 3).[20] Other authors like Lavery et al. (2010) argue that sponsors and investigators also need to discharge their obligations to address the conditions of background injustices. Wendler and Shah (2017, 9) dismiss this approach. They contend that concerns related to background injustices are important, but distinct from the concerns addressed in the context of (community) exploitation. More specifically, the ethical obligations of researchers and sponsors are narrower than obligations to mitigate unjust background conditions. The fair play model and, more specifically, my interpretation of community exploitation as free-riding on the efforts of communities, does not run into this problem. This is the case because the principle of fairness places agents under obligations in a pre-institutional context, which yet ignores the structural or institutional deficits in other sectors.

Second, I want to emphasize that I interpret Phillips' principle of fairness to be regulatory for "reasonably" just schemes but not necessarily "optimally" just schemes (Tosi 2018, 4). We may say that a jointly produced good must be at least worth the recipients' effort in providing it and presumptively beneficial (Klosko 1992, 39, 2005). In health research, the produced scientific knowledge with potential social benefits must be worth the recipients' effort in providing it and potentially beneficial to a host community. Here, the nature of benefits and obligations are tied to the outputs of the knowledge production. To ground fairness obligations, the fair play model demands that research is set up as a reasonably fair cooperative scheme. Without further specifying the content of fair benefits,[21] it is true that a community is *not* bound to support a highly unjust scheme, e.g., a scheme in which it is *ex ante* clear that communities are afforded an unfairly small part of the benefits that result from scientific knowledge. This may be, for instance, the case when the research question of a study is of no potential use for a community.

A "reasonably" fair scheme, then, makes a research enterprise justifiable and subject to fairness considerations. We may also contend that the moral wrong of "free-riding" comes by degree. Often, investigators and sponsoring agencies do not quite free-ride but rather "cheap-ride" on the efforts of communities. There is some latitude in the determination of when researchers and sponsors fully and fairly cooperate in a scheme of fair benefits, when they cheap-ride, and when they fully free-ride. Our moral condemnation for community exploitation should certainly depend on the degree of free- or cheap-riding.

Finally, my interpretive approach to community exploitation as free-riding on the efforts of communities conceptually matches other accounts of exploitation that have been put forward as critiques of Wertheimer (Mitra 2012; Wenner 2015). The emergence of obligations under the principle of fairness can help us understand on a conceptual level why research that does not adequately return benefits to communities can be considered exploitative. I thus offer an interpretation of community exploitation that emerges from the current literature and directly comments on what research ethics scholars have argued (Annas and Grodin 1998; Glantz et al. 1998; Mitra 2012; Snyder 2012; Wenner 2015).

Objections to the Fair Play Model and Replies

Here, I will reconstruct and reply to four possible objections to the fair play model. I am aware that there are many more objections, especially to a general theory of fairness or fair play (see Arneson 1982; Nozick 1974; Simmons 1979a,b, 2001). I cannot consider all of them and will choose the most pertinent objections to my major claim. The four objections address (i) the voluntariness constraint of accepting the reception of benefits, (ii) the membership problem of collaborative enterprises, (iii) the non-bindingness of the principle of fairness in other commercial interactions, and (iv) the moral and conceptual force of the social value requirement in research ethics. While the first three objections consist in very general arguments against the principle of (stakeholder) fairness itself, the last objection is directed more specifically toward its application to health research. I will argue that if we accept a theory of fairness or fair play, these problems remain challenges brought forward by anarcho-libertarians, but do not threaten my core idea of applying the principle of stakeholder fairness to health research.

Voluntariness

According to Hobbes, "benefits oblige" (Leviathan 11.7.11). There has been much discussion on how exactly obligations under the fairness principle arise. While many have only criticized the principle of fairness as groundwork for political obligations, Robert Nozick (1974, 90–5) argues that it fails as a moral principle in every context. Following Nozick, the academic discussion has been centered on the "voluntariness requirement" regarding the reception of benefits as a precondition for any kind of fairness obligation (Arneson 1982; Nozick 1974; Simmons 1979a,b, 2001), which has also been taken up in Phillips' interpretation of stakeholder fairness.

Nozick's (1974) libertarian objection in *State, Anarchy, and Utopia* is that the associative nature of a joint collaborative enterprise does not necessarily create obligations without voluntary, express consent. Hence, the obligation-creating feature at stake is not related to the reception of benefits but to consent. One of his most famous examples is the following:

> Suppose that your best way of getting exercise is by throwing books into people's houses, or that some other activity of yours thrusts books into people's houses as an unavoidable side effect. [...] One cannot, whatever one's purposes, just act so as to give people benefits and then demand (or seize) payment. Nor can a group of persons do this. (Nozick 1974, 95)

The book-thrusting example shows that bestowing benefits—Nozick believes that the recipient of a book indeed receives a benefit—without consent cannot lead to any type of obligation. Arneson's (1982, 618) example of a gift-giving association takes up Nozick's example and develops another point more clearly, as follows: Members of a gift-giving association refer to the principle of fairness when a justification is demanded for their forcing residents of the neighborhood to comply with the rules of the organization of gifts. By showering a neighbor with gifts, they attempt to create an obligation on the part of this neighbor to return gifts to the rest of the group. However, according to Arneson, such an associative venture does not automatically create the obligation to reciprocate in the gift-giving enterprise, even if gifts are voluntarily accepted.

Arneson (1982, 618ff) demonstrates that the gift-giving association and Nozick's book-thrusting example hint at what we understand as private (excludable) goods. They may be produced and distributed via a joint cooperative scheme, but the benefits attached to their consumption are exclusive. The crucial point is that a community is generally free to exclude a person not willing to cooperate with the rules of the gift-giving club. This is the case because the members of the club are free to carry on the scheme without forcing the participation of others. Then, the voluntariness condition becomes subsidiary: even voluntary receipt of a gift from the association, as mediated by its rules, does not necessarily generate obligations in the recipient. This means that if one is presented with a gift from the associated neighbors, one has the option to accept or reject and still does not bear an obligation to reciprocate.

There are two possible replies to this challenge. First, Klosko (2005, 2014) thinks that the creation of obligations based on a theory of fair play lies in the fact that one ought to obey a cooperative scheme as long as the scheme is worth its costs, presumptively beneficial, and fair. Once these conditions are fulfilled, we can assume that individuals rationally want to have the goods at stake. If people do not want them, we shall consider them *ex hypothesi* nonrational or for some other reason mistaken. An interesting clarification of Klosko's (2005) framework is that goods must be worth their costs. For this purpose, he introduces *essential goods*, a set of goods that each individual is reasonably expected to want because they are pertinent to a reasonably good life.[22] Thus, part of the reason why obligations under the principle of fairness can be bestowed on individuals is owed to the indispensability of the provided goods, as it is the case regarding many public goods like national defense, public health and so forth.

Klosko's argument can be read in a very Kantian spirit, as it would be irrational to sustain a state of nature in which those essential goods are lacking.[23] At the end, Klosko argues that Nozick's examples, in which cases are construed around relatively negligible goods and values, serve as "rhetoric means" (Klosko 1992, 39). He claims that the mere receipt of benefits is not morally binding in the case of private (mostly trivial) goods, such as gifts, and also in the case of public radio stations and public address systems (to name some of Nozick's public good examples). Klosko claims that his own account applies to cooperative schemes that provide essential (public) goods. This includes health research as one essential source of important public health benefits (Klosko 2005, 34).[24]

Second, Phillips (1997, 57–8) offers another objection to Nozick regarding the voluntariness constraint. He argues that Nozick's examples suffer from a misinterpretation concerning the use of the fairness principle. The person Nozick finds exempt from obligations of fairness may indeed be exempt from such obligations. The core intuition is the following: in Nozick's examples (e.g., the book-thrusting example), a collaborative scheme is built up around benefits recipients (like the receivers of the books) without their involvement; such recipients are not cooperators in the scheme in the appropriate sense but "innocent bystanders." Such a person has not acted in a way that could be interpreted as having willingly and voluntarily accepted the benefits in question. It is important to recall that there is a distinction between "accepting" and "receiving" benefits. An individual accepts a benefit (i) if she has tried and effectively obtained the benefit or (ii) if she takes openly and consciously the benefit (Simmons 1979b, 108).

As a general rule, acceptance of some benefit implies steps taken to receive or procure it (Klosko 2014, 160; Simmons 1979b, 324). For instance, the person in the book-thrusting example does not try to get the benefit or does not take the benefit willingly and knowingly (Phillips 1997, 58; Simmons 1979b, 108). Thus, the example does not give rise to special obligations of fairness. In turn, the important idea conveyed by the orchard example (Section "The Principle of Stakeholder Fairness") is that there are many cases in which fairness obligations arise precisely because individual parties openly and consciously take advantage of benefits. Phillips (1997, 58) holds that this is the case for any activity, and this would, importantly, certainly include the reception of gifts in a gift-giving association, where benefits are voluntarily accepted.

Regarding Klosko's and especially Phillips' argument, the voluntariness requirement does not pose a major problem for the justification of fairness obligations borne by researchers and sponsors. International researchers and sponsors are voluntarily involved in international research projects, meaning that they try (i) to effectively obtain benefits from a joint venture and (ii) take them openly and consciously, as they drive the initiation of a research project in a host community. What about the community members? I argued above, following Rawls (TJR, 100), that we do not necessarily need to show that community members are placed under fairness obligations if our aim is to show that researchers and sponsors are morally obliged to comply with fairness constraints in a collaborative scheme. Fairness obligations primarily fall on privileged agents who fully and willingly accept benefits on the basis of cooperation. Nevertheless, we may say a few more words about the status of communities.

Admittedly, unless community members voluntarily serve as research subjects, they do not give express consent, as they are forced by institutions to pay taxes in order to provide infrastructure or to make a tested drug available in the health system. However, drawing on Klosko's (2005) approach, the social value of epistemic research outputs can arguably be considered as an essential good with a public character (see Klosko 2005 on research and public health, Klosko 2014). It would be irrational to forgo such a good from a community's perspective. Therefore, the enforcement of a collaborative scheme under fairness constraints can be justified. Importantly, community members are, however, only placed under fairness obligations if the collaborative scheme is reasonably just (Phillips 1997; Van Buren 2001; Klosko 2014). This presupposes, for instance, a working health system in which community members have a fair opportunity to effectively access medicines, e.g., via health coverage. Members from LMICs and certain socioeconomic classes cannot be asked, e.g., to pay tax money or to serve as research subjects if only the rich have access to health care (see Hughes 2012, 628). Fair play demands that a considerable cross-section of community members contribute to and benefit from health research. Community members owe fairness obligations to one another, which might be discharged by, for instance, implementing just national tax and health systems.

The Membership Problem

The principle of fairness is commonly challenged by the so-called "membership problem" (Gilbert 2006, chap. 1), which is directly related to the voluntariness requirement. Philosophical anarchists, such as Nozick (1974) and Simmons (1979a, b, 2001), find it hard to justify the claim that individuals *qua* members of a certain collaborative scheme should be charged with obligations. Simmons' (1979a) critique is that Nozick's (1974, 94–5) examples are all examples in which an "outsider" has some benefit thrust on her by some cooperative scheme to which she is not tied (like the book-thrusting case). As we saw in the past section, philosophical anarchists think that these benefits do not bind under the principle of fairness, if they are not voluntarily accepted. So, we may summarize this position as follows: consent obligates, benefits do not. However, according to Simmons, voluntary participants in the cooperative scheme ("insiders") are candidates for being obligated under the principle of fairness to do their fair share. But outsiders are not bound even though they may benefit, as they do not consent.[25] In other words, membership of an identifiable group does not make someone automatically a participant, even in the case when one cannot avoid receiving certain benefits. Thus, the principle of fairness can only bind insiders that are already collaborating individuals, as they have accepted the fair terms of cooperation. This eventually renders the principle of fairness for stakeholder identification superfluous.

Defenders of the principle of fairness have tried to counter this objection. It would be too cumbersome and not fruitful to enter the debate.[26] However, let me outline two possible stances on this. Drawing on Klosko (2005, 2014), we can identify "insiders" to a collaborative scheme as not only *all (voluntary and involuntary) contributors* but also *all (voluntary and involuntary) beneficiaries* of a collaborative scheme. An individual becomes subject to a collaborative scheme in which (positive) externalities are created through the reception of benefits of a presumptively essential good, independently of her consent. Current scholars in research ethics, and most notably Levine (2008), have advanced the thesis that the social value of knowledge in research is an essential part of everyone's life due to the potential (public) health benefits each of us receives from the knowledge creation. Just think of the advances in disease prevention, antiretroviral therapies, or disease control through vaccines, to mention some of many possible examples.

But there may be another way of identifying stakeholders. Stakeholders are first and foremost all cooperators that qualify as such in an interaction, based on the requirements formulated by the principle of stakeholder fairness. Cooperators contribute to a scheme of mutual advantage and presuppose restrictions on each party's liberty in a significant way in order to achieve a collective end. As Phillips (1997) shows in the orchard example, non-cooperators in an initial situation are put under an obligation to become contributors as soon as they willingly benefit from a collaborative scheme. This raises an important issue. The social value of knowledge in research and the attained positive externalities frequently accrue to people outside the communities where research projects are conducted. For instance, especially citizens of HICs willingly make use of the knowledge produced in offshore research trials, as they can access drugs that have been tested elsewhere, thanks to functioning health systems in their countries, without bearing significant burdens of research. Taking individuals in other countries into consideration would considerably extend the number of "insiders" within the scope of fair play. Interestingly, Barry (1982, 229) made an attempt to introduce the principle of fairness to the debate on *global justice* as having a "potentiality for underwriting a certain amount of redistribution from rich to poor insofar as one practice that might be regarded as prospectively beneficial to all concerned would be the practice of helping those in need." I will scrutinize this point in more detail in Chapter 5.

Other Commercial Interactions

The fair play model relies on the foundations of stakeholder theory in business transactions (Phillips 1997; Van Buren 2001), including a variety of practices, such as trade, manufacturing, and other business operations. Here, one major critique may be that fairness obligations cannot strictly be extended to *background* contributors, such as community members understood as citizens of a host country. Consider the following two cases:

> *Sweatshop Labor.* Company B produces shoes in a LMIC country and pays worker A an exploitative wage. This has significant positive externalities, which are enjoyed by beneficiaries in HIC countries, as, for instance, cheap shoe prices due to the offshored production sites. The common view holds that B bears an obligation to pay its workers a fair wage, which leads to increased shoe prices in HICs. However, B does not necessarily hold an obligation to share benefits with the wider community.
>
> *Unfair Trade.* Trader B buys coffee beans from farmer A in a LMIC country. Trader B would be able to pay a higher "fair" price but prefers to retain a greater profit margin and pay A an exploitative price. A common view is that this creates obligations to the poorer country. However, it is also commonly held that these obligations can only be that trader B pays a fair price; they do not entail that trader B shares benefits resulting from trade (e.g., part of her profits), with the community A belongs to.

The key concern of the "common view" in both *Sweatshop Labor* and *Unfair Trade* is that the community A belongs to cannot be established as an ethical subject or stakeholder in a business transaction. Communities may have a single claim as stakeholders: party B ought not to place a net burden on the country where she (it) operates (Hughes 2012). However, Phillips' (1997) principle of fairness establishes stakeholders as cooperators that restrict in some relevant sense their liberty; that is, they contribute to a just scheme of mutual benefit where potential free-riders exist. I added that weak unanimity demands that all stakeholders have a minimal participatory intention, that is, an individual role to contribute to a joint end can be identified. A second dimension of fair play and stakeholder fairness concerns the extent of fairness obligations or fairness as a regulatory norm in relation to the burdens cooperators bear.

To partly oppose the common view that communities cannot be established as ethical subjects, let me start with the *Sweatshop Labor* case. Communities restrict their liberty by providing positive background contributions (by bearing an increased tax burden for the public goods and facilities needed, and by bearing opportunity costs) in a scheme that is thought to produce an economic benefit. I assume that the ultimate aim of the shoe production is economic benefit, not the good itself (which makes it distinct from research, where I consider the production of socially valuable knowledge to be the joint end, even though economic benefits may also be produced). Even if community members do not completely consciously or willingly contribute to this goal, they nevertheless contribute by playing a causal role and bearing burdens for the creation of economic benefits together with B and A. Institutions usually recognize these contributions as such.

Despite this rather weak notion of unanimity, we may nevertheless say that communities are stakeholders in a cooperative scheme in which fairness obligations arise, as suggested by Phillips (1997) and Van Buren (2001). Regarding the extent of these fairness obligations, it is possible that compensatory (tax) payments for positive background contributions, compliance with adequate and ethically acceptable work, safety, and environmental standards by the operating company are enough to comply with fairness obligations. My point is: these activities to return benefits can be sufficient to comply with Phillips' (1997) principle of stakeholder fairness, as background contributors do not bear burdens to the same extent as workers, CEOs, and other direct contributors do. Reciprocated benefits are expected to reflect burdens of relevant stakeholders and their (background) contributions, but not more than that.

Unfair Trade may be more ambiguous. At the first glance, one can argue that prices resulting from trade spill over to the local community to which the producer belongs, for instance, because farmer A employs other community members. In some way, the farmer's use of resources and public goods also indirectly conditions the transaction between A and B. Nevertheless, it is difficult to perceive interaction or mutual restriction, and thus a shared collaborative scheme between trader B and the community A belongs to. Benefits from the use of resources, workers, and benefits resulting from the use of public goods do not accrue to B but are reflected in the price offer of A, who is required to act as a fair cooperator in her community. Then, it seems to be morally right that B (only) pays a fair price in the transaction with A without returning further benefits to other community members.

Nevertheless, even though trader B does not bear obligations to community members, she may bear a duty to abstain from transactions with farmer A that in some way *harm* others. Harm would result from a transaction, e.g., when human rights are violated or when the local economy or society of A is harmed in some other relevant sense. Examples include the sale of toxic waste and weapons to local merchants in LMIC communities or narcotrafficking. Importantly, the general duty not to harm is different from special fairness obligations, or the obligation to return fair benefits within a collaborative scheme. Moreover, B may bear a duty to abstain from taking advantage of structural injustice, comprising political and social injustices and structural poverty prevailing in LMIC contexts (Malmqvist 2013; see also Chapter 6). When B pays A an unfair price, she takes advantage of the unfair background conditions that enable her to engage in unfair transactions. However, "taking advantage of background injustice" is a moral wrong relative to the transaction between B and A and should, again, not be confused with fairness obligations to other community members.

I hold that the examples of other commercial interactions (*Sweatshop Labor* and *Unfair Trade*) do not rule out the possibility that researchers and sponsors have special fairness obligations toward community members in a wider sense. Indeed, *Unfair Trade* cannot be reconstructed as a collaborative scheme between communities and traders. Nevertheless, *Sweatshop Labor* demonstrates that stakeholder fairness includes background contributors in collaborative schemes regarding business interactions. The case furthermore shows that the extent of fairness obligations depends on the relative contributions by community members (Phillips 1997), given (a minimum of) weak unanimity in a collaborative scheme.

The Social Value Requirement in Research Ethics

Allan Wertheimer (1999, 2011, 2015), an ardent follower of the libertarian position, argues that the social value of knowledge has no normative grounding. I already outlined the details of his argument in Chapter 2: the social value requirement is neither necessary nor sufficient to prevent exploitation, and (at least) privately funded research should not be taken to be an unethical use of public tax money. If we think that Wertheimer (2015) is right about this, the following objection will pose an important challenge to my account.

My main argument in this chapter revolves around what I call the justification requirement. I explain why researchers and sponsors are placed under obligations to cooperate fairly with host communities by appealing to the fact that researchers, sponsors, research subjects, and communities jointly aim to produce a good of (fair) *mutual benefit*, i.e., knowledge with social value. What is missing in my argument is, however, a justification for the social value requirement. The problem here is that health research with either low social value or no social value lacks a just end and does not yield collective benefits from which (a large number of) contributors potentially benefit. Thus, even if my arguments were sound for research with socially valuable benefits, research showing an insufficient or no social value would not bind researchers and sponsors to "strong" fairness obligations, at least not under my outline of the fair play model. In light of the discussion in the previous section, we may, however, contend that research without social value yet counts as an economic activity—with a weak degree of unanimity, but sufficient to establish the conditions for a wider collaborative scheme.

In what follows, I will argue that we can still assume a (relatively) high degree of unanimity among community members, researchers and sponsors, and research subjects in view of their joint end to produce socially valuable knowledge. Before proceeding, let us think of a clear example of research with low or no social value. "Me-too" drug trials are commonly cited as a type of research that lacks social value. Such trials study drugs that are similar to already approved treatments in terms of their indication, side effects, administration, and costs; their development has no potential additional benefit to future patients (Wendler and Rid 2017).

Interpreting the literature and usual practice in research ethics, I have so far presupposed two things. First, I took it for granted that the social value of knowledge *ought to be* the central good produced in research (following the CIOMS-WHO guidelines 2016; Emanuel et al. 2000; Levine 2008; Mitra 2012; Wendler and Rid 2017; Wenner 2015, 2018a), which means that research projects without social value, should be excluded from legitimate research activities. Second, I assumed that socially valuable knowledge is in fact the central good in research and so places agents under fairness obligations.

Regarding the first point, I explained that most scholars and research ethics committees adhere to strong reasons not to approve research that lacks social value. Some of these reasons are beyond the intentional exposure of research subjects to risks (Emanuel et al. 2000, 2004; Jonas 1969; Levine 2008) and the argument that tax income has to be reasonably spent (London 2012). Additionally, research needs to foster and maintain public trust (Holzer 2017; London 2012) and researchers' integrity (Wendler and Rid 2017).

Furthermore, explaining the basic idea of research, Wenner (2018a) notes that "[t]he primary justification for the social value requirement lies not in the ethics of free and fair transactions but rather in the goals of the clinical research enterprise and the nature of its impacts on society" (Wenner 2018a, 29). This justification transcends other reasons, such as the exploitation of individual research subjects, the misuse of valuable tax money, individual integrity, or even public trust. Research is more than the instantiation of a single clinical study; it should be interpreted as a long-term and overarching activity for the good of humanity. As suggested by Levine (2008), research ought to generate significant value in *all* our societies to be ethically acceptable as to turn the Kantian concern that subjects are used as means for knowledge gain into an obligation of humanity to support and encourage research. In other words, socially valuable knowledge is the ultimate "just cause" of research.

My second point is that I consider research to be socially valuable from an empirical stance. Empirical evidence highly suggests that (even private) health research generally rests on the expectation that it will produce socially valuable knowledge, that is, a social surplus. Furthermore, Wendler and Rid (2017, 83) make the point that roughly one-third of clinical research is publicly funded, and the remaining two-thirds is still dependent on public investment. Scarce resources usually underlie public control and are normally directed toward the cure of diseases, disease eradication, and prevention.

Importantly, the issue here is not so much whether a study yields social value *per se*. Rather, we want to know to what extent clinical trials need to produce socially valuable knowledge that accrues to future patients of *host communities*. One of the major concerns in international research is that people abroad benefit much more from the generated knowledge than host communities. But if I am right, the rare study without *any* social value does not pose an important objection to my account resting on the social value requirement in health research.

Concluding Remarks

In the past chapters, I have criticized the application of Wertheimer's transactional account to fair benefit-sharing and community exploitation in international health research. Transaction-specific fairness remains a widely defended ethical groundwork in normative models, such as the economic model. In this chapter, my aim has been to reinterpret fair benefit-sharing and community exploitation under the fair play model. To do this, my point of departure consisted in demonstrating that research is best interpreted as a joint collaborative scheme among researchers, sponsors, research participants, local health authorities, communities, and other stakeholders with the joint end to produce mutual benefits, i.e., socially valuable knowledge.

So far, I have outlined the moral groundwork of fair benefit-sharing and community exploitation. I have not yet made a clear statement about the relation of exploitation to structural injustice (Chapter 6); neither have I yet specified what the content of fair benefits and fair procedures and mechanisms of benefit-sharing may be (Chapter 7).

5

Cosmopolitanism and the Extension of Fair Benefit-Sharing to Other Agents

The Global Scope of Fairness in Research

Since clinical research and the consumption of pharmaceuticals are globalized, we need to ask to what extent agents who benefit from offshored health research ought to return benefits to (specific) host communities. The basic premise of benefit-sharing is that, as a matter of justice, those who contribute to scientific research are owed a fair return. It immediately suggests that agents other than investigators and sponsoring agencies who benefit from research in LMICs naturally turn into free-riders. These "other" agents are mostly populations from HICs.

The history of ideas in both political theory and research ethics reveals that cosmopolitan normative models specifically target the affluent world by conceptualizing (distributive) justice as a global concern. A rigorously cosmopolitan perspective has not yet been considered in this book despite its prominence in the current research ethics literature. This chapter makes a decisive step toward the inclusion of affluent agents other than researchers and sponsors who benefit from international health research under a cosmopolitan framework. To state it upfront, my discussion of cosmopolitanism serves the completeness of normative models put forward to address the fair treatment of host communities. I do not suppose that cosmopolitanism—that regulates (distributive) justice on a global (systemic) scale and relates to the realm of universal duties—makes a contribution to what I specifically frame as "fair benefit-sharing."

Keeping this in mind, the focus of this chapter is twofold. I first ask in Section "Cosmopolitan Approaches to International Health Research" whether cosmopolitanism is somehow able to address the fair treatment of host communities by including duties of agents in a global perspective. To do that, I will outline cosmopolitan approaches widely known and defended in international research ethics: capability-based models, rights-based models, and models based on imperfect duties. In Section "Critique of Cosmopolitan Models in International Health Research," I point to specific critiques brought against these cosmopolitan models. Here, I will not try to discredit cosmopolitanism *per se*, as this would require a more in-depth discussion of cosmopolitanism and global justice and eventually hugely exceed the focus of this work. Rather, I aim to clarify that the *use* of cosmopolitan models to account for community-specific obligations is inappropriate. I will argue against the use of cosmopolitan models, as the realm of universal cosmopolitan duties in health research cannot ground special obligations of fairness.

The second part of this chapter investigates the scope of the principle of stakeholder fairness, rather than focusing on cosmopolitan duties. More specifically, Section "Cosmopolitanism and Its Limits Reconsidered under the Fair Play Model" will analyze whether the principle of fairness gives rise to special obligations of fair benefit-sharing borne by affluent agents other than researchers and sponsors. I will argue that special obligations of fair play indeed have a global reach. This depends on the inclusion criteria stated in the theory of fair play. Interpreted within the fair play model, direct beneficiaries of benefits resulting from research, being potential free-riders, can be placed under fairness obligations.

Cosmopolitan Approaches to International Health Research

As the word "cosmopolitan" implies (Greek *kosmopolitês*, "citizen of the world"), cosmopolitans believe that all human beings, regardless of their political affiliation, are (or should be) citizens of a single community (Kleingeld and Brown 2013). However, the label "cosmopolitan" has been used to describe a wide range of theoretical positions. Here, it would be too cumbersome and outside the focus to depict the major debates within cosmopolitanism.

Nevertheless, I would like to outline some important clarifications relevant to cosmopolitan theory that have so far been defended in the debate on (global) justice in health research. To start with, this chapter first focuses on cosmopolitan approaches that seek to establish the justificatory grounds for distributive justice—some benefit transfer from the global rich to the global poor.

Furthermore, it is useful to distinguish between *moral* and *political* cosmopolitanism. Moral cosmopolitanism makes no claims about the desirability of global institutional structures. It is important for moral cosmopolitans that all human beings are units of equal moral concern and should respect one another as such. The basic claim underlying moral cosmopolitanism is that morally arbitrary factors should not affect what individuals owe to each other. These morally arbitrary factors comprise, e.g., gender, race, and nationality (Nussbaum 1994). This leads moral cosmopolitans to the claim that we have strong universal duties of justice with a global scope. Authors defending moral cosmopolitanism can be found among utilitarians (e.g., Singer, Unger), Kantians (e.g., O'Neill, van Hooft, Consani et al.), or Aristotelians (e.g., Nussbaum) and approaches combining these (Heilinger, Held and Maffettone). All seek to establish duties of justice or virtue toward the needy. There are also approaches associated with "cultural" cosmopolitanism, which hold that individuals should engage with, learn from, and respect diverse cultures while maintaining a sense of shared humanity. This perspective emphasizes moral concern for people beyond one's own community or nation, and yet insists that cultural differences ought to be acknowledged rather than assimilated or erased. Thinkers such as Kwame Anthony Appiah argue that one can remain deeply rooted in one's own cultural traditions while still embracing cosmopolitan ethical responsibilities toward others (Appiah 2006; see also Zhang 2017).

In contrast, political cosmopolitans differ from moral cosmopolitans because they focus on institutions rather than on duties toward individuals. Again, there is support for a wide range of proposals, including a centralized world state, a global federal system with limited coercive power, and a more modest global institutional reform. Recent philosophical discussions on international political arrangements have been led by Charles Beitz, Thomas

Pogge, Kok-Chor Tan, and more lately Japa Pallikkathayil, and many others. These positions are often, but not necessarily, opposed to a strong "non-relational" view, arguing that principles of distributive justice are grounded in relationships through global institutions (Beitz 1979).

Some of the most pertinent cosmopolitan approaches in research ethics have focused on an institutional re-design of global research institutions. Banerjee et al. (2010) global "Health Impact Fund" and Ballantyne's (2010a) "Global Research Tax" are examples of proposals intended to tackle an unfair distribution of benefits and burdens resulting from pharmaceutical research at a global institutional level (for an extensive discussion, see Chapter 7). All these approaches are pertinent to the literature of global research ethics because, I will later argue, they have inspired the most contemporary literature on research ethics.

Indeed, to state it upfront, these approaches must be understood as emerging from a normative paradigm that has been partly critiqued by contemporary literature on "white saviourism," itself grounded in broader postcolonial critiques. The dependence of many LMICs on foreign research and imported medicines is a legacy of colonial extraction, structural adjustment policies, and restrictive intellectual-property regimes—a vulnerability particularly exposed by the COVID-19 crisis. From the perspective of global justice, what LMICs are owed is the transformation of pharmaceutical sovereignty from a political slogan into a sustainable, locally anchored capacity (see Holzer et al. 2023a; Finkel et al. 2022; Luna and Holzer 2025; Mulumba et al. 2025).

Unfortunately, the full scope of this critique lies beyond the purpose of this book. Nevertheless, as we will see in Chapter 7, some mechanisms of fair benefit-sharing will intersect with the post-colonial cosmopolitan critique, particularly in relation to community engagement in global health research. In the following sections, I will outline selected cosmopolitan approaches in health research ethics that have been proposed earlier to guide benefit-sharing, specifically justifying the flow of benefits from the affluent to the communities where research is conducted. These approaches are normative models that extend moral duties to, generally speaking, affluent agents, including citizens from HICs, researchers, and sponsors. Cosmopolitan normative models comprise both the cosmopolitan theories they are grounded in and proposals for how to discharge cosmopolitan duties in practice. I will examine examples of capability-based, rights-based, and imperfect duty cosmopolitan approaches for the fair treatment of host communities.

To state it upfront, this is a very incomplete list that contains very different approaches within the cosmopolitan paradigm. While some of the approaches clearly adhere to moral cosmopolitanism (London 2005; Millum 2011; Pratt and Loff 2013, 2014), others start from a political or institutional point of view (Pogge 2002, 2005a). My decision to include the normative models I have chosen is due to their significance and prominence they have gained in the debate on global justice in health research. These approaches were among the first to systematically connect cosmopolitan theory with the moral challenges of global health research, including benefit-sharing and the risk of exploitation when drugs are tested in economically disadvantaged communities in other countries. Importantly, these approaches continue to be discussed in the literature and have, for instance, been applied as theoretical frameworks during the COVID-19 pandemic. For this reason, I consider these approaches particularly worthy of discussion in light of my own development of the fair play model.

Capability-Based Approaches

There are two main approaches in research ethics that rest on what I will introduce as *capability-based* theories of justice. On the one hand, Bridget Pratt and Bebe Loff (2013, 2014) have developed what they call a "framework to link international clinical research to the promotion of justice in global health." On the other hand, Alex John London (2005; see London and Kimmelman 2008) has developed a framework that he calls the "human development approach," which addresses the links between medical research, human capabilities, and global justice. Even though there is no explicit reference to the "capability view of health" (Ruger 2004), London's (2005) general approach is related to the work of two of the most prominent capabilities theorists, that is, Amartya Sen (1981, 1999) and Martha Nussbaum (Nussbaum and Sen 1993).

Before outlining the two approaches, I would like to briefly describe their common theoretical fundament. Both models can be traced back to the "capability view of health" (Ruger 2004, 1075). In Ruger's framework (2008), health has a special moral importance due to its status as an end of political and societal activity. In her view, society has an obligation to maintain and promote health, as this rests on the ethical principle that Aristotle calls *human flourishing* or *well-being* (Greek, *eu̯dai̯monía*) (Ruger 2008, 7–11, chap. 2.1). Many aspects of health sustain all other aspects of human flourishing because, without being reasonably healthy, no other human functions are possible. The term *health capability* captures the moral importance of an individual's opportunity to achieve good health and to be free from escapable morbidity (Ruger 2008, 47f).

Ruger's health capability theory relies on the *human capability approach*, most prominently defended by Amartya Sen and Marta Nussbaum. Sen's (1999) account distinguishes human capabilities from other established approaches to ethical evaluation, such as utilitarianism (e.g., Singer) or resourcism (e.g., Dworkin), which focus on subjective well-being or the availability of means to a good life for an individual. In contrast, a person's capability to live a good life represents a set of valuable "beings and doings" (capabilities). While Sen (1999, 2002) has been mostly concerned with the practical implications for the evaluation of welfare politics,[1] Nussbaum (1990, 1993, 1997) is one of the most prominent philosophers who focus on a capability theory of justice based on Aristotle's legacy. According to Nussbaum (1990, 1993), "functioning" serves as an indicator of how people are doing and how they can exercise their freedoms and their practical reasoning faculty. Not only governmental but also global engagement is required to provide and secure the conditions, goods, nutrients, services, and basic rights to support human flourishing to a sufficient extent.

Pratt and Loff's Framework for the Promotion of Justice in Global Health through International Health Research

Pratt and Loff (2013, 2014) adjust Ruger's health capability paradigm to the context of international health research. They argue that the health capability paradigm "supports a universal duty to efficiently reduce shortfall inequalities in health from the optimal global level as determined by mortality and morbidity" (Pratt and Loff 2014, 388). Consequently, every individual is entitled to appropriate health care goods and services for prevention, diagnosis, treatment, and rehabilitation, which include appropriate environmental, social, and political structures that enable the individual's capability to be healthy.

Health research is supposed to undertake a very specific task to develop and optimize global health levels and to fill gaps regarding the responses of the worst-off host communities to local illnesses. Also, clinical research shall promote host communities' own research capacity and offer *post-trial benefits* (Pratt and Loff 2014, 390–2). These "obligations" do not only accrue to researchers and sponsors but to multilaterals, global institutions, citizens of HICs, and national governments (Pratt and Loff 2014, 389). In principle, states are the primary agents. However, when they are unable to fulfill their populations' health entitlement, "justice requires that global actors assist states to ensure their populations' health capabilities and build state capacity to do so" (Pratt and Loff 2014, 388; Ruger 2009). Obligations shall be allocated according to the functional requirements principle. This means that different agents are assigned obligations because the functions they typically assume make them particularly capable of fulfilling the obligations (Pratt and Loff 2013, 2014; Ruger 2009). In this sense, affluent actors, such as governments of HICs, researchers and sponsors, may carry major responsibilities.

Furthermore, under the label "research for health justice" Pratt and Loff (2014) put forward certain principles to regulate health research as well as corresponding implementation strategies:

- Community selection: Pratt and Loff suggest prioritizing the globally worst-off communities instead of seeking to do research on diseases prevalent in high- and middle-income countries. Host communities from which research subjects are recruited must have a large gap in health status relative to the optimal level, so that research can contribute to improving health among the worst-off.
- Capacity-building: In Pratt and Loff's view, health capabilities cannot be strengthened without adequate community capacity-building.
- Choice of health conditions: The investigated health condition should be a local concern, which means that major contributions should be made to the community's health status.

In a more recent paper, Pratt suggests, this time together with Hyder (Pratt and Hyder 2017), a scheme for fairly allocating resources to public health, health care, and health research. They make a case for public and private funders in HICs bearing an duty to spend benefits on nondomestic health research.

London's Human Development Approach

London's (2005, 2008; see London and Kimmelman 2008) human development approach emerges from a critique of the economic model. In the eyes of the human development approach, the economic model has been the best-developed approach in research ethics but lacks sufficient attention to the health needs and capabilities of the global poor. According to London (2005, 25), mutually advantageous bargaining represents "justice as mutual advantage." This view offers savagely exploitative outcomes, given that the bargaining power between researchers and sponsors on the one side and host communities on the other side are never balanced (London 2005, 25ff; London and Zollman 2010; see Chapter 3).

London's (2005) aim is to offer a model that makes explicit the links among health research, the social determinants of health, global justice, and human development. In particular, he thinks that a morally permissible division of labor and benefits "must strive to secure for individuals ... the 'fair value' of their basic capacities for welfare and human agency" (London 2005, 29). London claims that the economic model fails to address these basic capabilities of host community members and denies populations access to social health resources to which they have a moral claim.

London's framework appeals to us by taking the basic interests of the global poor seriously. This gains special importance because most of the avoidable mortality in LMICs is due to a few causes of disease for which effective interventions already exist (Jha et al 2002, 2036; London and Kimmelman 2008, 84). However, he notes that a normative model cannot be grounded in unmet *obligations* to host communities, as both are rooted in pre-existing relationships between sponsoring agencies (and researchers) and host communities. I similarly argued in Chapter 4 that the notion of distributive justice has serious shortcomings if it is grounded in obligations that arise from special prior relationships between host communities and agents and corporations from HICs. The problem is that these agents to do not necessarily have any prior normative relationships with research populations in the developing word.

Since London (2005) is aware of this potential critique, he neither presupposes any prior normative relationship between researchers together with sponsoring entities from HICs and host communities nor assumes that a research initiative would utilize any material, institutional, or human resources from the population. Rather, London grounds his approach in the *duty to aid* that is owed equally to all humans. London further specifies the cosmopolitan duty for affluent agents to aid as a duty to "create and sustain social structures that secure individuals' capacities for welfare and human agency" (2005, 32). In the context of health research, this duty spells out the conditions under which clinical research represents a permissible activity.

London calls his framework grounded in the duty to aid the *human development approach*. Research poses one valuable means for researchers, sponsors, and other affluent agents to discharge the duty to aid. This is accomplished by fostering appropriate basic social structures to guarantee community members the "fair value" of their most basic human capabilities. London argues (2005, 25) that because the health status of individuals is affected by political, social, and economic factors, the project of creating and sustaining the conditions that foster health requires a coordinated, multi-sectoral approach sensitive to these factors (see also Daniels 2008; Marmot Wilkinson 2003). This perspective regarding the role and function of international health research has a direct impact on the evaluation of clinical trials. Research is a permissible enterprise when it functions to expand the capacity of the basic social structures of a community to better serve the fundamental interests of that community's members.[2]

Pogge's Human Rights–Based Approach to a Global Health Research Reform

In this section, I will focus on Thomas Pogge's human rights–based approach to global health research. I will leave out other important and substantive human rights–based cosmopolitan theories (e.g., Barry 1982; Shue 1996) that identify a duty to actively promulgate and foster the human rights of the global poor (see Kime 2009, chap. 1). There is an impressive and substantive canon of literature on this, which I unfortunately cannot address within the scope of this work.

Pogge's theory differs from substantive human rights approaches, which present a human right as something that places us under certain constraints independent of social institutions. In contrast, Pogge advocates an institutional understanding of human rights, which he conceives as a human meta-right to an effective legal right to X. He thus constructs a human right as follows:

> The postulate of a human right to X is tantamount to the demand that, insofar as reasonably possible, any coercive social institution be so designed that all human beings affected by them have secure access to X. A human right is a moral claim on any coercive social institutions imposed upon oneself and therefore a moral claim against anyone involved in their imposition. (Pogge 2002, 46)[3]

Governments are required to ensure that all human rights are incorporated into its fundamental legal text, observed and enforced through an effective judicial system (Pogge 2002, chap. 1). This conception of rights leads Pogge (2002, 47) to the claim that institutions can be blamed for not fulfilling or underfulfilling human rights, rather than for violating them.

What I find most interesting in Pogge is, however, not his conceptualization of human rights per se but rather two other aspects of his theory. First, Pogge makes an interesting conceptual move regarding the duty toward the global poor, as he converts a positive duty to foster and to sustain human rights into a negative one.[4] The foundation of his theory is indeed rights-based, but reveals, beyond that, a duty-based approach that justifies institutional reforms. This point shall be of significance in this chapter, which is concerned with the plausibility test of a cosmopolitan demand to attain fair community treatment in international health research.

Second, Pogge explicitly applies his theoretical framework to the context of health research and argues, based on his theory, that a practical proposal for attaining greater health justice is needed. He proposes, together with

Banerjee and Hollis (2010), a global reform in international health research by introducing the "Health Impact Fund," which is thought to be an innovative incentivizing mechanism for research and development of pharmaceutical products to address the health needs of the global poor (Pogge 2005a; see also Holzer 2016; Pogge and Laukötter 2013). For now, I will leave the practical proposal aside; I will revisit it in Chapter 7, which is dedicated to the principles, procedures as well as implementation mechanisms of fair benefit-sharing.

To understand Pogge's conceptual foundations for a global institutional reform in health research, we should examine his book *World Poverty and Human Rights: Cosmopolitan Responsibilities and Reforms* (2002).[5] Pogge's argument for a negative duty to promote human rights relies on two normative premises (see Sonderholm 2012, 367): first, that there is a morally significant distinction between actively causing poverty and failing to prevent it; and second, that global justice involves a primary focus on negative duties, which are minimal constraints on conduct that worsens the situation of others (Pogge 2002). Pogge's main argument concerns the second premise: it is false that affluent members of developed countries are not actively causing severe poverty in developing nations. They cause poverty in virtue of imposing a burdensome global order on the global destitute that deprives them of the fulfillment of basic human rights (Sonderholm 2012, 367ff). Here, Pogge finds himself in stark contrast to the positions of other authors, who propagate a positive, or at least not a merely negative, duty toward the global poor (see Shue 1996; Singer 1972; Temkin 2004; among others). According to Pogge (2005a, 5), negative duties are compelling in the sense that they imply duties not to expose people to life-threatening poverty and further duties to shield them from harms for which we are actively responsible. However, this is what is happening in the international context: harm is caused by the affluent.

Pogge's negative duty has frequently been conceptualized as a "duty of rectification" that is incurred by all citizens of affluent nations whose policies and international activities have contributed to the plight of the developing world (London 2005, 30; Wenner 2015, 78). Regarding global health, Pogge claims that global institutions have serious repercussions in developing countries because access to life-saving medicine is impeded through high prices attained under intellectual property protections (e.g., under the current

TRIPS agreement).[6] According to Pogge, the affluent world could avoid these harms by simply reforming its global institutions, such as the World Trade Organization, the World Health Organization, and the International Monetary Fund. More specifically, the developed world could agree to a greater opening of their markets and refrain from demanding the strict protection of intellectual property (Pogge 2005a; Pogge and Laukötter 2013).

In "Testing our Drugs on the Poor Abroad," Pogge (2008) explicitly directs the focus of justice in international health research on the rectification of global injustice and the role developed nations play. Here, the sole focus on "fair research" overshadows the importance of global reform. Pogge, like the capabilities thinkers, rejects the claim that *volenti non fit iniuria* (Latin, "to the willing, no injury is done")—a phrase that can be attributed in particular to the economic model (Wertheimer 2011).[7] People deprived of the most basic resources and health outcomes are violated in their human rights even if they consent to negotiated benefits and to hosting research. The fact that pharmaceutical research into drugs and vaccines is incentivized under the current rules has created various bilateral agreements and clinical trials that can be questioned on ethical grounds.

Imperfect Duty Approaches

To state it upfront, my division between capability, rights-based, and duty-based approaches may not be compelling in the sense that the first two categories also come along with duties—either positive duties, such as Pratt and Loff's (2014) duty to foster human flourishing, London's (2005) duty to aid and to foster human flourishing, or a negative duty not to harm others or violate their human rights (Pogge 2002). However, there is a difference between these and what I call *imperfect duty approaches*.[8] The framework I will refer to with this label focuses on duties, or differently put, takes the duty-bearer as a starting point. This duty-bearer has an *imperfect* duty rather than a *perfect* duty matched by counterpart rights.

Onora O'Neill (1996) is one of the most prominent authors to have extensively criticized what she calls rights-based approaches for reasons having to do with their too narrow scope and minimal reach in the institutional international order. What cosmopolitans like O'Neill suggest is to focus on imperfect duties of virtue, rather than on institutionalized perfect duties that belong to the realm of *justice*. In Section "Rights without Duties, Duties without Rights," I will outline in more detail the reasons for this claim. Bearing O'Neill's reconstruction of duties in mind, I will outline one exemplary imperfect duty account along these lines defended by Joseph Millum (2011), who applied the duty of beneficence to international health research.

Millum's Imperfect Duty of Beneficence

Millum (2011) defends an imperfect duty of beneficence in the context of international health research. This "weaker" form of cosmopolitanism may face less critique regarding O'Neill's concern against perfect duties (see Section "Rights without Duties, Duties without Rights"). In "Post-Trial Access to Anti-Retrovirals: Who Owes What to Whom?"[9] Millum addresses, among other principles, duties of beneficence that require us to increase the welfare of others. He identifies one major source of these duties: there is a "limited" (I suppose he means *imperfect*) duty to improve other people's welfare, which he calls the "duty of beneficence" following Kant (Millum 2011, 152). Millum (2011, 152) states that this imperfect duty can be discharged in any way and anywhere: "by volunteering at the local homeless shelter, by campaigning to clean up the Chesapeake Bay, or by babysitting my neighbor's children." In the context of health research, a duty of beneficence could be discharged in the form of benefit-sharing with host communities, but this would be only one of many ways to fulfill such a duty.

Nevertheless, it should also be mentioned that Millum (2011) identifies a second source of general duties of beneficence, that is, a "duty of rescue," which requires us to provide urgent assistance to others where we can do so at a morally insignificant cost (see also Singer 1972, 2009). Millum (2011, 152f) explains that the duty of rescue can be framed as a duty of *specific beneficence* (see Beauchamp and Childress 2001, 171). He thinks that the duty of rescue could give rise to *special obligations* of researchers and sponsors toward research subjects who urgently need help and would otherwise die (e.g., when research subjects are HIV positive, and they are not in the possession of the appropriate drugs). It is certainly possible to argue for a broader scope of the duty of rescue, e.g., to members of host communities. Peter Singer (1972, 2009) is one of the major advocates of a general duty of rescue, which he illustrates with the famous example of the child drowning in the pond. This makes sense when the costs of rescue are comparatively low. For instance, there are valuable normative models that expand the duty of rescue to additional care for research participants and other community members (see Merritt et al. 2010; Richardson 2012, 15).

However, I suppose that Millum would object to the claim that researchers and sponsors have a duty to rescue (a duty of specific beneficence toward) community members other than research subjects with whom they do not stand in direct relation. Here, the problem is not that a duty to rescue would require a direct relationship. Nevertheless, the costs of providing drugs or other benefits to (many) community members are definitely higher when researchers and sponsors are not in a position in which they directly reach out to community members. It also seems that researchers and sponsors could discharge their duty to rescue in any community, not necessarily the one hosting their research trial. Thus, it might be more in line with Millum's framework to focus on the duty of general beneficence to address the duties of researchers and sponsors toward host communities. Addressing a host community's health needs, post-trial availability of drugs, and other benefits could be a way for researchers and sponsors to discharge their imperfect duty of beneficence. But as Millum notes, this is not the only way of discharging this duty.

Critique of Cosmopolitan Models in International Health Research

The core request of the outlined cosmopolitan theories for health research concerns the assignment of cosmopolitan duties to other, presumably affluent, agents. These agents are either thought to assume direct responsibilities toward poor communities or are identified as the agents responsible for reforming global institutions to render international health research more just. In Section "General Objections to the Foundational Arguments of Cosmopolitan Theories," I will sketch some common critiques of (especially) moral and political cosmopolitanism, with a focus on the proposals outlined above in health research ethics. Since the debate on global justice is too broad, I will leave out major debates in the contemporary literature. Moreover, I do not want to purport to side with or to reject cosmopolitanism but rather include these critiques for purposes of presenting a complete discussion.

In Section "Cosmopolitanism and Special Obligations in International Health Research," I will put forward an argument against the use of cosmopolitan models to explain obligations toward host communities, as these approaches do not ground *special* and *perfect* obligations borne by researchers, sponsors, and other affluent agents and owed to specific host communities. In short, my main argument is that cosmopolitan theories in international health research can show that affluent agents, including researchers, sponsors, and citizens of affluent nations, bear cosmopolitan duties—and even that these agents bear a great part of such duties—but they do not give rise to special obligations toward the *specific* communities where research is conducted. Thus, I do not put forward a direct critique against cosmopolitan duties *per se*. I solely contend that the realm of universal cosmopolitan duties cannot ground special obligations of fair benefit-sharing.

General Objections to the Foundational Arguments of Cosmopolitan Theories

I will briefly outline some critiques of central concern against cosmopolitanism to provide a complete panorama of the theories (and their critiques) cosmopolitan normative models in health research are based on. I will solely focus on arguments that apply to the frameworks I outlined in Section "Cosmopolitan Approaches to International Health Research."

The Statist Objection to Non-relational Cosmopolitan Theories

What the accounts defended by Pratt and Loff, London, and Millum have in common is that they postulate universal and non-relational duties that ought to be discharged in the context of international health research.

The "statist critique" is strongest when used to reject *non-relational* principles and theories of global justice. Under this label falls a wide range of different frameworks and theories that oppose non-relational cosmopolitan accounts. As previously explained, relational approaches to justice hold that justice is grounded in features of the social, political, or institutional relationships that prevail between moral agents. Our positions relative to other people are justice-apt features that give rise to duties or obligations that we owe to one another. Prior to such relationships we do not have any, nor can we have any, duty or obligation. Relations are important components of the architecture of justice because individuals themselves share goods and cooperate together to achieve particular ends, or stand in a common relation to a particular institutional structure so that some form of equality applies to them (Miller 2001b, 26; see also Kime 2009, chap. 3).

Blake (2001), Miller (2001b, 2008), Walzer (1994), and Rawls (TJ, TJR) have most notably offered relational accounts that define the scope of justice to be within the borders of nation-states. In their view, the affiliation with nations has intrinsic and fundamental moral significance (Kime 2009, chap. 3). Miller, for instance, argues that "circumstances of justice," meaning the conditions that must be in place before principles of justice can apply, are linked to bounded societies, effective institutions, and the possibility of change. His theory of global justice is fundamentally different from his view of justice in nation-states. He argues that we should understand global justice in a way that takes account of large differences between the domestic and international context: global justice does not involve principles of distributive justice, as it is not linked to strong bounded societies and effective institutions. The statist critique denies that there are strong cosmopolitan duties of (distributive) justice on the grounds of a missing relational "entanglement" of agents operating in a global context. (Kime 2009, 70; Miller 2008, 21). This critique can be applied to the frameworks put forward by Pratt and Loff, London, and Millum, as far as duties to address the global poor involve resources from HICs.

Critique of Pogge's Negative Duty

The statist critique is weaker when applied to Pogge (2005a), assuming that he can make a convincing case for a negative duty arising from sufficient global interdependence of actors, i.e., a global *relational* scheme. However, Alan Patten (2005) has offered an extended criticism of Pogge's negative duty approach

(Sonderholm 2012, 365). He claims that Pogge makes an unconvincing case for the underlying causes of global poverty. According to Patten, there are factors other than the unjust global institutional order that underlie global poverty. According to Jorn Sonderholm (2012), this critique has been taken up by several authors, such as Cohen, Gilabert, and Risse. Here, I will briefly mention some selected lines of argument found in Sonderholm's (2012) work.

Pablo Gilabert (2005) objects to Pogge's concept of a negative duty because he thinks that he essentially turns a positive duty into a negative one. Violating a negative duty—namely, a duty not to harm X—cannot mean that one fails to improve the situation of X as much as possible (Gilabert 2005, 542; Sonderholm 2012, 377). Mathias Risse criticizes Pogge on different grounds. He intends to show that the global order does not harm the poor if one adopts the baseline of comparison that Pogge suggests. Maybe to our surprise, we observe an international trend indicating that the global order has led to improvements of the status of the global poor over the years. Risse says that the world order is not unjust but at most "incompletely just" (Risse 2005, 10; Sonderholm 2012, 377).

Joshua Cohen (2010) explains that Pogge's framework is underwritten by a very strong claim—that most of the global poverty problem could be eliminated through minor modifications in the global order that would lead to only slight reductions in the incomes of the affluent (Cohen 2010, 19). However, there is reason to be skeptical: perhaps *only some* global poverty could be eliminated by changes in global rules (Cohen 2010, 26), or perhaps poverty is only induced by domestic causes, such as corruption, and the power abuse of local politicians and officials (Cohen 2010, 23).

Rights without Duties, Duties without Rights

O'Neill (1996) has extensively argued in *Towards Justice and Virtue* that cosmopolitan duties do not make sense when these duties are not institutionalized. She claims that social justice liberals mistakenly fear that imperfect duties would not be sufficient to protect the poor from deprivation (O'Neill 1996, 143f). Theories motivated by these concerns are quite often based on rights, like Pogge's account. Likewise, the health capabilities approach in international research calls upon the notion that affluent agents owe to the global poor the fair value of their human capacities. The idea is that the global poor possess a right, which then creates and matches a corresponding duty of the affluent to rescue them from poverty and poor health. To understand O'Neill's further critique, let us have a look how she links those rights and duties:

> The deontic links between agents arise because the deontic status of an act can be characterized both from the perspective of the agent and from the perspective of others with whom the agent stands in various sorts of relationship. For example, if A owes B an act of a certain type, or its omission, B will be entitled to such performance or omission by A; if B is entitled to have A perform or omit an act of a certain type, A will have an obligation so to do. These and other deontic relationships … allow for systematic arguments that link various practical requirements. (O'Neill 1996, 127)

When *deontic links* cannot be established, meaning that a rights-holder cannot be matched with a corresponding duty-bearer, O'Neill sees no point in claiming a right. Rights are then merely "rhetoric" and cannot be claimed, waived, or enforced. It is the task of institutions to identify rights-claimers and duty-bearers in order to establish deontic links. In her view, justice is exactly about these *perfect* duties, or, about rights and duties that can be matched. There are indeed universal duties—held by all and owed to all—such as liberty rights and the legally enforced duty to respect them. However, regarding positive rights, such as welfare rights, it is not at all clear whom we may identify as an obligation-bearer. If critics are right that Pogge's attempt fails to reformulate a positive duty to promote welfare rights to subsistence as a negative and universal duty, then O'Neill makes a very valuable point.

Now, consider the context of international health research: Who is actually to blame for not fulfilling the right to adequate health levels, health capabilities, or human rights in poor countries? Following O'Neill's account, it is arbitrary to identify researchers and sponsors or any citizen of an affluent country as duty-bearers on cosmopolitan grounds. This is the case because cosmopolitan duties are not adequately and compellingly institutionalized in global health research.

There are many powerful agents out there and it is not clear who owes what to whom in exact terms. Cosmopolitan accounts are very vague regarding the specification of the agents who are responsible for initiating global reform. Without this specification, cosmopolitan frameworks remain mostly rhetoric. Moreover, if all affluent global citizens bear a cosmopolitan duty to rescue, aid, or rectify, it seems arbitrary that specific affluent agents like researchers and sponsors are the primary responsible actors, again given that cosmopolitan duties are not adequately institutionalized and borne by all agents, not some.

I already mentioned that O'Neill (1996) has a solution in mind for how we can cope with the global justice problem in global anarchism: while perfect universal duties are held by all and owed to all, imperfect universal duties of charity are held by all, but owed to none because there is no counterpart right (obligations without rights). These duties are duties of character and virtue and do not presuppose deontic links between right-holders and duty-bearers. O'Neill most notably mentions the duty of charity we bear toward our fellow human beings.

It seems Millum's (2011) duty of beneficence applied to international health research comes close to O'Neill's virtue ethics account, meaning that it can be conceptualized as a duty of virtue, as a strict deontic link is not needed. However, as I will argue in the next section, an imperfect duty does not help us get to special obligations of fair benefit-sharing owed to specific host communities. If we want to justify any possible (future) institution or binding legal framework for fair benefit-sharing, we must identify *justified deontic links*. In addition, an imperfect duty of beneficence could never provide adequate criteria for specifying "how much" an affluent agent A owes to an impoverished agent B, as the realization of imperfect duties is beyond the realm of (distributive) justice (O'Neill 1996).

Cosmopolitanism and Special Obligations in International Health Research

As I mentioned before, this section is not concerned with presenting a criticism of cosmopolitanism but only an objection that the outlined cosmopolitan approaches cannot ground special obligations, that is, obligations owed to specific host communities and not generally to the global poor. Cosmopolitanism in international research ethics generally offers comprehensive approaches to how a cosmopolitan duty may be realized in international health research. Then, research is just one possible way to discharge the duty of aid, beneficence, or rectification.

Here, I want to point to a great inconsistency cosmopolitan frameworks face when they postulate *community-specific* special obligations on grounds of universal duties. Especially the capability-based frameworks seem to face this critique. As Pratt and Loff (2014) suggest, capacity-building should be provided to host communities, and the medical intervention under testing should be a specific response to the health conditions of the research community. I am tempted to interpret these demands as explicit postulations of special obligations, especially if they are meant to be mandatory in every health research project. In my view, this can hardly be justified on grounds of a general duty.

We might argue that under a cosmopolitan framework, researchers and sponsors are required to share their benefits not with the host community exclusively (including rich community members) but with the global poor in general. It should be justifiable, within a cosmopolitan framework, to ask a sponsoring agency to engage actively with multiple communities in community capacity-strengthening, post-trial access, responsiveness to health needs (of global concern), philanthropic revenue-sharing or donation to agencies that develop aid projects in low-income countries, or participation in the effective altruism initiative.

My objection is, however, that obligations to give *more* benefits to (or to address health needs and capabilities of) a particular host community can only be grounded in special relationships between researchers, sponsors, affluent nations, and host communities. If special obligations grounded in special relationships are not present, as in the case of cosmopolitan (universal) duties, there seems to be an "outsider objection" (see Jeske 2021). The outsider objection says that special obligations run up against a complaint made by people similarly affected by global injustice and poverty: it is not clear why researchers, sponsors, and other affluent agents are obliged to do more for a certain host community compared to any other community from LMICs that is also affected by global injustice.

Admittedly, cosmopolitan duties can be a point of departure on the basis of a quasi-consequentialist argument according to which whoever is in a good position to discharge general duties should do so. So, researchers and sponsors may be in a good position to discharge a cosmopolitan duty to help a specific community, as Pratt and Loff (2014) or Wenner (2015) advocate. However, this does not rule out my objection that the same agents could obtain knowledge from one community and transfer the benefits, i.e., medicines, to another (poorer) one.

Cosmopolitanism and Its Limits Reconsidered under the Fair Play Model

My argument in the previous section is simple: cosmopolitan frameworks alone cannot justify special obligations toward communities, such as obligations of benefit-sharing. As I argued, the reason for this lies in the missing *deontic links* of cosmopolitan accounts. On the one hand, non-relational cosmopolitan accounts grounded in a (perfect or imperfect) duty of aid or beneficence do not address justice as redistributive fairness in collaborative schemes and hence lack a theory of fair reciprocity. On the other hand, relational cosmopolitans cannot show that fair benefit-sharing or the demands of distributive justice need to be community-specific.

We may, however, sustain that non-relational cosmopolitan approaches, such as the ones by Pratt and Loff, London, and Millum make important points regarding the general role of health research in fighting global poverty. Relational approaches by Pogge (2002, 2005a) (see also Banerjee et al. 2010) have made progress in this debate with a global reform proposal related to global distributive justice. Indeed, much of this is very valuable and should be further advertised and developed.

Here, I specifically want to explore whether my fair play model of Chapter 4 is a valuable alternative to moral and relational cosmopolitanism in research ethics.[10] The question is to what extent the fair play model can reach out to, generally speaking, agents from the affluent world. My strategy is as follows: I already showed that we can justify special obligations of researchers and sponsors toward host communities on the grounds of the principle of stakeholder fairness. Now, my aim will be to show that obligations under the principle of fair play[11] accrue to other agents in the international sphere. This gives my approach (and the concept of fair benefit-sharing more broadly) a cosmopolitan orientation.

The Membership Criterion for Joint Enterprises Reconsidered

In the following, I will explain why affluent agents (other than researchers and sponsors) bear special obligations to host communities when they profit from offshored clinical trials. My claim is that the principle of fair play and its adaptation to stakeholder fairness accounts for obligations borne by beneficiaries in the affluent world. Socially valuable knowledge in the realm of health care frequently accrues to people outside the communities where research projects are conducted. Citizens and agencies from HICs are able to access the knowledge and drugs that have been tested elsewhere thanks to functioning health systems in their countries. Thus, they accept benefits created by others.

As explained in the previous chapter, stakeholders are first and foremost cooperators that qualify as such in an interaction, based on the requirements formulated by the principle of stakeholder fairness. Cooperators contribute to a scheme of mutual advantage and accept restrictions on their liberty to achieve a collective end. However, as Phillips (1997, 59) convincingly argues, non-cooperators in an initial situation are put under an obligation to contribute if they willingly accept benefits from a cooperative scheme. Moreover, the membership criterion and thus the focus of fair play relates to the beneficiaries and not primarily to the contributors (Klosko 2005, 2014).

In Chapter 4, my point of departure was joint agency, meaning that I tried to identify and focus on possible contributors, thus making clear that research is a collaborative enterprise. Beneficiaries like affluent individuals and agencies abroad (mostly from HICs), even though not part of the initial cooperative enterprise, are not only passive bystanders who are involuntarily "exposed" to public benefits from the knowledge production in LMICs. They rather willingly *accept* (and not only receive) benefits because they make use of the produced knowledge—for example, when they implement tested drugs in their health care system (see Klosko 2005, 2014; Phillips 1997; Simmons

1979a, b). Agencies like the US Food and Drug Administration do that when they license and allow for the commercialization of medicines or other medical interventions tested abroad. Citizens consume knowledge created abroad by accessing an intervention. Nevertheless, we should not forget that beneficiaries in the affluent world are arguably themselves contributors to the collective end of research when they pay either privately or with their tax money for the drugs tested in offshored trials. They show participatory intentions insofar as they are contributors and beneficiaries once the benefits from drug testing abroad are made available in their own countries. Then, these agents ought to contribute fairly to the joint enterprise.

We should also add that beneficiaries other than researchers and sponsors are not only located in HICs but often belong to poor communities, or even the host community itself. This is the case when some individuals have the means to effectively take advantage of socially valuable knowledge and others (of the same community) do not. This is frequently due to significant income disparities caused by background injustices. It is also frequently the case that privileged individuals in non-ideal contexts characterized by background injustices do not adequately contribute to the development and improvement of national health systems. Moreover, governments in LMICs bear morally binding obligations beyond benefit-sharing in health research, e.g., the obligation to redistribute resources fairly and to respect socio-economic human rights, such as the right to health. Thus, community exploitation should not be narrowly conceived as committed solely by the affluent in HICs and by pharmaceutical companies. Rather, it is useful to draw a more realistic picture that includes other agents, such as government representatives of host countries that may equally participate in, or at least do not hinder, exploitative practices (see Barugahare 2016; Barugahare and Lie 2015).

To emphasize an important strength of the extension of the fair play model to other affluent agents, it is reasonable to assume that deontic links are established, as obligation-bearers and benefit-claimers can be identified within joint ventures, even though this link is not necessarily institutionalized. Obligation-bearers are all those individuals who have accepted the benefits from cooperation and owe a fair return. Benefit-claimers are all those individuals who have contributed to a joint enterprise and have a legitimate claim on fair benefits that ought to be returned to them. In health research, community members who contribute to a health research trial can rightly claim benefits from beneficiaries, such as researchers, sponsors, people living in HICs and other agents, who bear corresponding fairness obligations.

The Fair Play Model and International Health Research

Following my claim that a joint enterprise can be established across borders, let us examine our exemplary historical case, the Havrix trial (Chapter 1). The research study, sponsored by the U.S. Walter Reed Army Institute of Research and SmithKline Beecham, was designed to test a hepatitis A vaccine for the US military and travelers from Western countries. In accessing the vaccine, these wealthy agents from wealthy countries benefited from the social value of the knowledge generated during the trial. The same applies to the example of dengue vaccines: Western companies such as Sanofi produce socially valuable knowledge by developing vaccines, while these vaccines are not sold to the communities where the trials are conducted (Tully and Griffiths 2021).

It should be noted that the US military has been a leading proponent of vaccine development throughout its history. The reason for this is simple: one of the most cost-effective ways to maintain health of military personnel (across a wide range of geographical locations) is by vaccinating (Ratto-Kim et al. 2018). To this end, the Department of Defense (and more specifically the US Army Medical Research and Material Command) sponsors trials to test potentially beneficial malaria vaccines around the world, e.g., in Kenya, Mali, and also at research sites in the United States (Graves and Levine 2006, 53). In *Battling Malaria: Strengthening the U.S. Military Malaria Vaccine Program*, Graves et al. together with the Committee on U.S. Military Malaria Vaccine Research offer a program review of trials actively undertaken and sponsored by the Department of Defense. These trials are thought to facilitate deployment abroad in malaria-endemic areas and thus, to actively promote and maintain national security (Graves and Levine 2006, 5).

We may therefore argue that part of the obligations to contribute to research should be borne by its beneficiaries, namely travelers, the military, or more generally, individuals who can access a tested drug as patients. Regarding the Havrix trial, there are other countries that benefited from the research study, even though they were not involved as sponsoring countries in the research process. For instance, Havrix is a registered prophylactic vaccine in many European countries. Several European pharmaceutical companies hold licenses for different indications of the Havrix vaccine, which are frequently covered by national health insurance systems.[12]

It moreover seems that benefits are directly traceable not only in the Havrix trial but also more generally in a lot of drug research: they mostly fall upon members of rich countries that are able to make good use of the knowledge gained in offshored research. One particular point of health research worth mentioning is that no country rich enough to access the created knowledge and the medical interventions under testing can be excluded from potential health benefits. Thus, socially valuable knowledge necessarily has a global reach. In consequence, I believe that the social value of international health research trials, which provide the foundation for medical progress, is a global quasi-collective good that can be potentially accessed by individuals, agencies, and countries that are in possession of adequate means (e.g., sufficient health and technology infrastructure, skills, resources, and capacity) to make effective use of the knowledge. To use the knowledge means to transform it into a (public) health benefit. This arguably gives rise to obligations under the principle of fair play on the part of all beneficiaries: (affluent) countries and citizens, as well as researchers and sponsors.

Eventually, considering that all contributors to a research trial are legitimate right-claimers in the sense that they have a right to get the fair value of their contribution, we can easily make a case that all affluent agents benefiting from international health research owe much more to host communities than is suggested by current practice. The important point is that there are special obligations by the affluent in play. The question about how these fairness obligations should be discharged (through licenses, a global research tax, etc.) remains a different concern related to the question about the appropriate principles and mechanisms of fair benefit-sharing (see Chapter 7).

So far, the outcome of my analysis resembles Pogge's cosmopolitan analysis: the affluent world benefits from international health research in poor countries (Pogge 2002, 2005a), which generates obligations to change current practices. However, there is a slight but significant difference between my own account and those of other cosmopolitans like Pogge. First, my fair play account does not hinge on a global institutional critique because it is a pre-institutional approach, meaning that the reception of benefits does not necessarily presuppose an institutional structure.

Second, where cosmopolitans try to apply a general cosmopolitan duty "top-down" because they ground special obligations in a general duty (like Pratt and Loff 2014), I advocate a more plausible justification for benefit-sharing, namely, that special obligations arise from a benefit-creating joint enterprise. The argument remains the same as in Chapter 4: we can presume that affluent beneficiaries in other countries participate in a presumably just research activity with the participatory intention to either produce and/or make use of socially valuable knowledge. Beneficiaries of the social value of research are aware that they draw benefits from the activity and moreover evidently accept benefits when they turn the respective benefits into improved health services, treatment supply, national security, and so forth, in their home countries. This creates the obligation to return a fair share to all contributors, including the community, research subjects, researchers, and sponsors, whose efforts have created socially valuable knowledge.

Third, the principle of fair play, i.e., stakeholder fairness (Phillips 1997), captures free-riding as a moral wrong that is committed when beneficiaries do not adequately contribute with a fair share of the costs to a joint activity, i.e., to the production of a good from which they benefit. Imagine a scenario in which a very rich country A tests drugs in its own territory. Country A neither implements drugs tested in poor countries into its national health care plan nor sends sponsors to foreign research sites. Now, imagine a second scenario in which country A tests drugs in LMICs. Cosmopolitan duties of beneficence or aid could easily make A subject to the duty to transfer benefits to poor countries due to A's capacity as a rich country to help the global poor. This is true even in the first scenario, in which country A never benefited from international health research.[13] A strictly *non-relational* cosmopolitan would probably claim that there is no moral difference between the two scenarios. Duties arising from beneficence or the capacity to aid are not necessarily grounded in the reception of benefits from the poor. However, the fair play model is able to explain and to identify a moral difference between the first and second scenarios.

The fair play model remains more precise in defining free-riders in the global sphere that benefit from the generation of the socially valuable knowledge produced by research. Citizens and health systems in wealthy countries frequently profit more from international health research as "opportunity free-riders" (*parasites d'opportunité*, Chauvier 2013, 200). These agents extract a recurrent or long-lasting benefit from the efforts of other agents, namely research participants and host communities, as well as sponsors and researchers. The effective use of new tested medicines is easier in high-income contexts with the means of working health care systems and infrastructure available. In turn, it is frequently the case that poorer countries get fewer benefits from the produced knowledge or at least take more time to benefit from medical progress (e.g., when generics of tested drugs are made available outside patent regimes, but years later). Moreover, global health disparities are even more reinforced when research questions are mostly tailored to the health needs of HICs (Hollis and Pogge 2008; Homedes and Ugalde 2016).

Fair Play and Global Justice?

In this last section, I will explain why I think that the literature is in line with the idea that the principle of fair play or stakeholder fairness can be obligation-creating, even on a global scale. In "Humanity and Justice in Global Perspective," Brian Barry (1982) suggests the principle of fair play to be a legitimate principle in the debate on global, especially distributive, justice:

> The principle of fair play has a potentiality for underwriting a certain amount of redistribution from rich to poor insofar as one practice that might be regarded as prospectively beneficial to all concerned would be the practice of helping those in need. … The principle of fair play would then hold that it would be unfair to be a free rider on a scheme of helping those in need by refusing to do your part when called upon. (Barry 1982, 229)

Thus far, my own account fits with Barry's formulation of the fair play principle in the international sphere. But eventually, Barry rejects the principle of fair play, offering the following reason:

> It is crucially important to notice, however, that the principle of fair play is conditional; that is to say, it stipulates that it is unfair to be a free rider on an actually existing cooperative practice, and that it would be unfair to free ride on other mutually beneficial practices if they did exist. But it does not say that it is unfair for a practice that would, if it existed, be mutually beneficial, not to exist. (Barry 1982, 231)

Barry here dismisses the principle of fair play[14] as conditional, meaning that it depends on already established cooperative enterprises, where it then grounds and regulates the distribution of benefits and burdens among different agents. But Barry wants to provide the foundations for a more general cosmopolitan framework that applies to the world beyond already established benefit-creating practices. The point he makes against the principle of fair play is sound in the sense that a theory of fair play cannot account for the duty of beneficence toward the worst-off.

The section "Critique of Cosmopolitan Models in International Health Research" of this chapter outlined that cosmopolitan theory (in international health research) potentially faces strong criticism. It is beyond the scope of my work to evaluate whether critics are right about the failure of cosmopolitan theory. However, what I want to point to is that the principle of fair play suggests an alternative way to justify at least *some* claims about global distributive justice. In this sense, the fair play model does not compete with cosmopolitanism. Rather, it reframes our commonsense morality regarding the global beneficiaries of international cooperative practices. Or, as Hobbes puts it, *benefits oblige* (Leviathan 11.7.11).

Let me dwell on one objection, which I call the "global distributive scheme" objection to my quite narrow interpretation of the principle of fair play. Readers could argue that I may end up claiming that the fair play principle accounts for a general duty of all affluent countries toward the global poor. This would be based on the assumption that the affluent world always free-rides on the positive externalities they receive from the global poor. The global institutional structure allows for free-riding and therefore constitutes a collaborative scheme. As we have seen, Pogge (2002) seems to allude to a similar argument. Likewise, Meketa (2014) argues that the global economy can be construed as a collaborative scheme in which the affluent willingly take advantage of the burdens on the global poor regarding the production of goods. If this is true, the fair play model collapses with some sort of political cosmopolitanism and I would not offer an alternative account to place the affluent under fairness obligations.

To address the "global distributive scheme" objection, I would like to point out that the principle of fair play, and particularly the adaptation and conceptualization of stakeholder fairness (Phillips 1997), does not apply to any kind of positive externalities other agents receive or, generally speaking, any kind of global spill-over effect resulting from national policies, global (institutional) relations, or the exchange of goods and services.[15] I argued that agents need to show at least weak unanimity, that is, a minimal participatory interest to either contribute to a collaborative scheme or to benefit from it in order to be considered a legitimate stakeholder (who can be potentially placed under fairness obligations). A participatory interest in a cooperative scheme can be reasonably assumed if an agent willingly accepts benefits, i.e., if she has tried and effectively obtained the benefit or if she takes openly and consciously the benefit (Simmons 1979b, 108). Many affluent countries and their citizens voluntarily accept benefits from socially valuable knowledge produced in LMICs when they use and implement new drugs in their national health plans or for the purpose of national security.

Following Barry's (1982, 233) argumentative line, there is, similarly, no genuine link between the principle of fair play and the redistribution of resources under a general cosmopolitan account. The principle of fair play does not apply to the sphere of global trade, agreements, and exchanges, based on the following reasoning:

> [I]t seems to be that trade [or other global relations and institutions], however multilateral, does [do] not constitute a cooperative scheme of the relevant kind. Trade, if freely undertaken, is (presumably) beneficial to the exchanging parties, but it is not, it seems to me, the kind of relationship that gives rise to duties [obligations] of fair play. To the extent that justice

> is involved it is, I would say, justice as requital, that is, giving a fair return. Justice as fair play arises not from simple exchange but from ... the provision of public goods that are collectively enjoyed (parks; defense; a litter-free, or unpolluted, environment; and so on). (Barry 1982, 233)

Barry offers a "public goods" argument to dismiss the concern that the fair play principle might ground a general obligation of distributive justice on a global scale. Obligations of fair play arise from the enjoyment of collective benefits where some agents potentially free-ride. Even though Phillips' (1997) conceptualizes stakeholder fairness irrespective of whether public goods are involved,[16] we may nonetheless say, as I have mentioned, that socially valuable knowledge, as an informational good, is at least quasi-collective[17] in the global sphere. At least countries rich enough to access and make use of the produced knowledge can easily free-ride on the collective benefit attached to socially valuable knowledge. The point is that HICs with a functioning health system and affluent individuals can easily access drugs and other interventions and treatments tested in LMICs. Depending on the tested intervention, researchers and physicians from HICs may also have the technological and the infrastructural means to access merely informational goods related to relevant study results and data produced abroad. Thus, knowledge implying enormous potential health benefits is easily accessible and usable for the majority of the developed world.

But again, isn't the whole world benefiting from the social value of biomedical research—even though benefits might vary depending on the relevance of a given treatment to a particular country and its access to that treatment? Is socially valuable knowledge produced in international research a global collective or even public good[18] no one can (completely) be excluded from? This rests on the assumption that at least some of the health benefits created through research are nonexcludable, such as immunization and disease prevention. Indeed, we may bear some examples in mind, such as the historical example of research done on the smallpox vaccine. Eventually, research and development resulted in the eradication of smallpox, which benefited citizens from poor and rich countries alike. I agree that it is very difficult to stipulate how much of the generated benefits accrue to an individual or an individual country compared to others. In such cases, it is impossible to trace every benefit flow, and to identify all beneficiaries and cost-bearers.

Still, I would like to set the "public goods argument" aside. Fair play, at its minimum, holds that where the reception of benefits is significant and essential, we may interpret this reception as *acceptance*, that is, some beneficiaries try (i) to effectively obtain benefits from a joint venture and/or (ii) take them openly and consciously (Simmons 1979b, 108; Phillips 1997, 57–8). Thus, where benefits from knowledge gain can directly be traced and contributors and beneficiaries identified, special moral obligations of fair benefit-sharing are *prima facie* justified.

Controversial cases and the public good discussion aside, many research trials show that it is not difficult to identify and trace back beneficiaries and cost-bearers of socially valuable knowledge produced in international health research trials. Returning once again to the much-discussed Havrix trial, the funding scheme, which was primarily supported by the US Department of Defense, suggests that the United States expected considerable benefits for its own country and its citizens, rather than for the host.

Concluding Remarks

My motivation in this chapter was to seek a normative model that assigns obligations to affluent beneficiaries in health research, in addition to researchers and sponsors. To do this, my strategy was divided into two major steps. First, I critically analyzed well-known cosmopolitan approaches that have been foundational to the ethics of global health research, examining whether cosmopolitanism can adequately account for this type of inquiry. I argued that cosmopolitan approaches cannot offer a valuable foundation for community- specific special obligations. This does not pose a fundamental challenge to cosmopolitan approaches in health research but undermines its relevance for the concept of fair benefit-sharing, as proposed under the fair play model.

My second line of argument concerned the "cosmopolitan" reach of the principle of fair play. I here agree with Barry that the principle of fair play can be applied to the international sphere, if done correctly. Since I interpret socially valuable knowledge as an essential informational good that can easily cross borders, I argue that any relevant beneficiary and potential free-rider on knowledge produced in international research is placed under fairness obligations. Affluent countries and their citizens are frequently major beneficiaries of the health knowledge produced in trials that are conducted in the developing world when they get access to drugs tested abroad. I argue that if we can make a convincing case that affluent agents and countries sufficiently and willingly benefit from the fruits of such research, they owe a fair share in return to the primary contributors, most notably, the host communities.

6

The Fair Play Model and Non-Ideal Theory: Accounting for Structural Injustice within a Theory of Exploitation: Reply to Fundamental Objection (ii)

The Moral Importance of Structural Injustice

In Chapter 3, I argued that one characteristic of purely transaction-specific accounts is that the concept of exploitation remains unrelated to its structural context. This has furthermore led to the common belief that researchers with their sponsors (and other agents, such as high-income countries profiting from research) are not responsible for remedying structural injustice. Wertheimer's (1999, 2008, 2011) theory defending this position seems to prevail in the standard literature related to clinical research (Emanuel et al. 2004; Emanuel et al. 2008; London 2005; Malmqvist 2013; Mitra 2012; Snyder 2012). Most notably, representatives and defenders of the economic model, such as Wendler and Shah (2017) and Emanuel (2008), sustain:

> [E]xploitation is a micro-level, not macro-level, concern. ... We should not confuse problems of distributive justice with problems of exploitation. Certainly macro-level distributions of resources can influence exploitation, but the actual exploitation is separate. Furthermore, while people may feel exploited and may claim to have been so based upon historical events, the ethical evaluation of exploitation does not depend upon a feeling or past injustices. Exploitation is about the fairness of an individual exchange. (Emanuel et al 2008, 93)

The aims of this chapter are as follows. First, I want to inquire what role (if any) the factor of structural injustice plays for the correct understanding of exploitation.[1] Second, I want to offer a new conceptual account that makes structural concerns a salient component of both *transactional* exploitation and *community* exploitation framed within the fair play model. My rationale is to demonstrate that even if we accept (transactional and community) exploitation as a phenomenon separate from structural injustice, we can and should still account for background injustices as a serious and impactful moral concern. Third, I want to inquire into the ethical and practical implications of my account for the case of international health research—notably, the moral concern to remedy structural injustice.

Before proceeding, I would like to make two clarifying remarks. First, proceeding from transactional models, and most notably the economic model, exploitative transactions can concern either individual research participants or communities. As I outlined in the past chapters, my main interest is dedicated to understanding how communities are exploited and how obligations of fairness arise toward communities in international health research. I have also argued that it is futile to follow the economic model and to frame community exploitation in transaction-specific terms. However, this chapter focuses on another moral dimension transactional models fail to account for, namely, the structural context in which unfair transactions take place. Thus, I will start by discussing the conceptual connection between *transactional exploitation* and *structural injustice*. Note that my attempt to account for community exploitation outside the transaction-specific focus by introducing a framework of cooperation under the fair play model similarly leaves out concerns of background injustice. Here, I, however, leave the concept of "community exploitation" aside until Section "Fair Play Model, Structural Injustices, and Community Exploitation," in which the connection between community exploitation and background injustice is deliberately made.

Second, when I focus on the relation between transaction-specific exploitation and structural injustice in health research, I mean to address voluntary and mutually advantageous and yet exploitative interactions—in short, mutually advantageous and consensual exploitation (see Wertheimer 1999, chap. 4; see also this work, Chapter 3). To keep it simple, I would like to introduce a standard case we find in the literature in which research subjects are exploited. This case reconstruction mimics frequently discussed research studies performed under a "double standard" (Chapter 2; Ballantyne 2005; Hawkins and Emanuel 2008; Malmqvist 2013, 2017). The following is Malmqvist's (2013, 558) case entitled *Clinical Trial*, which I prefer to rename:[2]

> *Double Standard Trial:* B suffers from a serious but treatable disease. Because she is poor and lives in a country that doesn't provide its citizens with basic health care, she lacks access to effective treatment. Pharmaceutical company A wants to conduct a clinical trial of a new and promising treatment for B's condition. In order to reduce costs and get more convincing results, A prefers to test the treatment against a placebo rather than against an existing active treatment. However, A predicts that a placebo-controlled trial wouldn't pass ethical review in a country where patients receive the existing treatment because it would require withholding that treatment from subjects who would otherwise get it. So, it is decided to conduct the trial in B's country instead. When approached with the offer to participate in the trial, B accepts. She is fully aware of what participation entails. She knows that she will only have a 50% chance of receiving the experimental treatment, but figures that a 50–50 chance is better than no chance at all. (Malmqvist 2013, 558)

The transaction-specific view on exploitation interprets Double Standard Trial as a paradigmatic case of wrongful exploitation because party A, the pharmaceutical company, takes unfair advantage of party B, the research subject.[3] In contrast, many defenders of a so-called "structural" account of exploitation argue that exploitation cannot solely be framed as a moral wrong within the narrow limits of a particular transaction between A and B, but must be considered as a direct consequence of background injustices (Cohen 1988, 1989, 1995; Ferguson and Zwolinksi 2024; Roemer 1996; Sample 2003; Wenner 2016; Young 2009, 2011; Zwolinksi 2012).

To develop my own account, I will proceed as follows. In Section "Mapping Competing Accounts of Exploitation," I will juxtapose the defenders and critics of structural accounts of exploitation that preceded Wertheimer's theory and those of more recent transaction-specific theories. Here, I will reconstruct the conceptual disagreement in the debate. I conclude that the critique urged by transactional theories toward structural accounts makes sense: exploitation cannot be treated as a *necessary* result of background injustice; nor is background injustice *sufficient* to explain exploitation. In Section "A New Framework for

Structural Injustice and Transaction-Specific Exploitation," I will nevertheless support the structuralists' main moral intuition—that background injustices matter in a defensible framework of exploitation—without animating the transactional critique. Therefore, I will introduce a framework based on a conditional probability argument that aims to conceptually link background injustice and a subset of exploitation I will call "systemic" exploitation. Part of my aim is to distinguish between systemic exploitation characterized as pervasive exploitative events that are probabilistically induced by background injustice, and "non-systemic" exploitation framed as exploitative events that remain uncorrelated to structural concerns.

In Section "Fair Play Model, Structural Injustices, and Community Exploitation," I will apply my insights from Section "A New Framework for Structural Injustice and Transaction-Specific Exploitation"—concerned with transaction-specific exploitation and background injustice and particularly the concept of systemic exploitation—to the framework of "community exploitation" under the fair play model. I argue that perpetuated structural injustice and its perturbing effect on international health research impact the accomplishment of fair cooperative networks and fair play. In this regard, I introduce the dimension of systemic community exploitation to complete the fair play model, filling the aforementioned gap. Section "Implications of Systemic Exploitation in International Health Research" addresses the implications of my account with respect to (i) the importance of background injustice to a theory of exploitation, (ii) moral responsibilities of different actors to prevent exploitation and to remedy background injustice, and (iii) the legal implications for permitting or banning exploitative clinical trials. Here, I will contend that that we can hold two ideas at once, namely, that responsibility for exploitation is broadly held, rather than borne solely by the agents involved in an exploitative transaction, and that structural injustices are nevertheless not determinative of exploitation.

Mapping Competing Accounts of Exploitation

The previous chapters focused on a very specific account of transaction-specific exploitation defended by the economic model, that is, exploitation understood as "transactional unfairness." I will now widen the discussion to more general transaction-specific and structural theories of exploitation. I will be particularly concerned with inquiring how these theories of exploitation relate to structural injustice. There are several different ways to account for exploitation and unjust background conditions: (i) purely transaction-specific accounts, (ii) intermediate transaction-specific accounts, and (iii) structural accounts of exploitation.

(i) Purely transaction-specific theories of exploitation. When referring to the general concept of transaction-specific exploitation, authors claim that there exists a morally wrong, nonreciprocal relationship between two individual agents A and B.[4] In the example *Double Standard Trial* the exploited party B voluntarily yields a net benefit from the exploitative transaction. However, what is morally wrong about such mutually beneficial and consensual yet exploitative transactions? A general answer is given by the following formula of transaction-specific exploitation (Wertheimer 1999, 232):

A wrongfully exploits B if A "takes unfair advantage" of B.

Philosophers disagree about the specific content of this formula. Some hold that the essential wrong of exploitation as "taking unfair advantage" consists in the violation of some norm of fairness (Mayer 2007; Valdman 2009; Wertheimer 1999, 2011). This is widely known as the "transactional fairness" approach, the theoretical core of the economic model. As I have explained, Wertheimer's theory of exploitation as transactional unfairness has had the greatest influence in research ethics (Emanuel et al. 2004, 2008; Hawkins and Emanuel 2008; Malmqvist 2013; Wertheimer 2011). In turn, the Kantian transaction-specific approach argues that exploiters wrong their victims not because they treat them unfairly but because they fail to respect them as persons (Sample 2003; Wood 1995). Others put forward what might be called the domination view, which conceives of exploitation as domination for self-enrichment (Vrousalis 2013, 2016). Finally, there are some authors who combine these approaches, holding that exploitation cannot be captured by a single interpretation of "taking unfair advantage" (Snyder 2012; Wilkinson 2003).[5]

These purely transaction-specific theories of exploitation have in recent years attracted many adherents. Exploitation framed solely in terms of an unfair transaction seems to replace the structural viewpoint. For the purpose of this chapter (concerned with the conceptual link between exploitation and structural injustices), my discussion of exploitation remains neutral among competing theories of transaction-specific exploitation. Wertheimer's and the economic model's theory of fair transactions according to the criterion of a fair market value is only one variant of the transaction-specific view.

(ii) Intermediate transaction-specific theories of exploitation. By "intermediate" transaction-specific theories, I refer to the views of authors who endorse transaction-specific theories of exploitation and also explicitly claim that there is an important empirical (even though not conceptual) relation between background injustice and exploitation. For instance, agent A in *Double Standard Trial* benefits from the inadequate health policies in B's country and especially B's lack of access to treatment, which makes it easier to recruit research subjects in an exploitative clinical trial.

Most notably, Erik Malmqvist (2013, 2017) has suggested that we can revive an account for the structural viewpoint that Wertheimer seems to ignore in his theory of exploitation, by re-introducing the moral wrong of "taking advantage of injustice." This concept captures not only the idea that A benefits from background injustice when she exploits but also that A helps sustain wrongdoing and an unjust state of the world (see Barry and Wiens 2016; Malmqvist 2013, 2017). In this regard, "taking advantage of injustice" poses a problem that often arises in transactions between economically powerful agents and the global poor.

When agents take advantage of injustice, they become *pro tanto* complicit in structural injustice.[6] *Complicity* can find expression in the following actions. In the first place, individual agents can act in response to structural constraints and possibilities and benefit from them, thereby constraining and enabling others to do the same. Furthermore, working complicitly with structural injustices signals to other future actors that turning structural injustices into profits is morally legitimate. By deliberately not repairing B's unjust circumstances (in the case of *Double Standard Trial*: giving her access to health care), the foreign agent A sends a message that those who ought to repair them (e.g., the governments of low- and middle-income communities) can continue neglecting their duties, as they will be neither sanctioned nor morally despised in any way.

(iii) Structural theories of exploitation. "Structuralists" argue that exploitation is not best understood as a feature of individual transactions but should instead be conceived as a structural phenomenon. Prior to Wertheimer's (1999) theory, almost all philosophical discussion on the concept of exploitation focused on a Marxist understanding. For Marx himself, exploitation was a feature of capitalism as a system and not primarily of individual transactions between capitalists and workers (Sample 2018; Wollner 2019; Zwolinksi 2012; Heðinsdóttir 2022; Gray 2020). While on the transactional view, cases like Double Standard Trial involve exploitation because B is unfairly, degradingly, or in some objectionable way exploited by A, the structural view reintroduces the broader social, economic, and institutional context wherein the transaction occurs to explain exploitation.

Broadly speaking, there are two ways of introducing structural injustice to the concept of exploitation. First, some structuralists claim that the contextual features of exploitation are intimately connected to structural inequalities that systematically render some groups of people liable to being taken advantage of by others. Yet, exploitation remains a transaction-specific concept, which is not necessarily induced by structural injustice (see Cohen 1988, 1995). Scholars considering themselves as "Neo-Marxists," such as Roemer (1996) and Cohen (1988, 1995), are proponents of such an account. Roemer, for instance, conceptualizes exploitation as an unjust asset flow that is the subordinate consequence of an initial distributive injustice. He therefore concludes: "exploitation conceived of as the unequal exchange of labour should be replaced with exploitation conceived of as the distributional consequences of an unjust inequality in the distribution of productive assets and resources" (Roemer 1996, 96).

Second, instead of taking structural injustice to be evidence that particular transactions within the context of those structures are exploitative, we may say that legal and economic institutions (the institutions that make up "the structure" itself) are themselves exploitative. Authors who put forward this view think that the "rules of the game" unfairly benefit one group of people to the detriment of another. Karl Marx believed that the economic and political institutions of capitalism were exploitative in this sense (Sample 2018). Contemporary philosophers have argued that social institutions, including traditional marriage, racist politics, and so forth, are exploitative insofar as they reinforce forms of inequality between men and women, or Caucasians and ethnic minorities (Manne 2017; Sample 2003, Ch. 4; Young 2009).

Why Transaction-Specific Accounts Prevail

In the following, I consider exploitation to be a transaction-specific concept, different from structural injustice. Generally speaking, the structural accounts I am primarily interested in, most notably represented by Roemer (1996) and Cohen (1988, 1995), contend that structural injustice is a *necessary* and *sufficient* condition for exploitation. This is not a causal thesis: it merely distinguishes just from unjust unreciprocated takings, by appealing to the moral legitimacy of the asset distribution (Vrousalis 2014, 153). Thus, exploitation is the consequence of an illegitimate distribution; or in other words, the legitimacy of the starting distribution determines whether an exchange is exploitative or not. On this analysis, when exploitation occurs, it is necessarily a result (or an "adverse effect") of illegitimate background structures, and the existence of such structures is sufficient to explain the exploitative character of the exploitative transactions that occur within them. Otherwise put, structural injustice is determinative of exploitation: for instance, researchers and sponsors can only be exploitative in their relationship with research subjects with the implication that the (global) research system itself must be overthrown.

Transaction-specific accounts oppose this strong conceptual connection between exploitation and background injustice. Wertheimer (1999), Valdman (2009), and Vrousalis (2013, 2014, 2016) have repeatedly argued that the structural account does not hold for many cases of wrongful but mutually consenting and beneficial exploitation. This means we can easily find cases of exploitation that abstract from structural concerns:

> *Antidote.* Person B is bitten by a rare poisonous snake while hiking in a remote forest. His death is imminent. Fortunately, another hiker, A, happens by and offers to sell B the antidote ... Though it retails for $10, A insists that he will accept no less than $20,000. Since B would rather lose his money than his life, he accepts A's offer. Here A wrongly exploited B. Indeed, this is about as clear a case of wrongful exploitation as I can imagine. (Valdman 2009, 3)[7]

If we accept that *Antidote*[8] presents an example of exploitation, the transaction-specific position seems to make an important point, namely, that structuralists illegitimately abstract from the personal wrongdoing exploiters commit in transactions when making structures the locus of moral concern. This attacks the structuralist idea that exploitation persists even without ill-will on the part of individuals who participate in exploitative systems. I concede that the general critique urged by transaction-specific theories toward structural theories makes sense: background injustice is neither necessary nor sufficient for exploitation. Also, exploitation as depicted in *Double Standard Trial* or *Antidote* needs to be framed as a moral wrong specific to a transaction, as reducing exploitation to unjust structures avoids the moral liability and individual responsibilities of the transacting parties.

Why Structural Concerns Matter

Many authors accept the transaction-specific view precisely because of the critique of structuralism suggested by *Antidote* (Malmqvist 2013, 2017; Zwolinski 2012). The transaction *itself*, these thinkers maintain, must have problematic features. Likewise, exploitative research is problematic because it is reasonable to assume that researchers and sponsors have the possibility to conduct fair trials. I think the structuralist intuition lingers, however, even in our evaluation of such cases: transaction-specific theories cannot account for the fact that background injustices make it easier, or even "tempting," for some to take advantage of others in a disrespectful way (Malmqvist 2017), even if they are not necessary or sufficient to explain the exploitative nature of such transactions.

Purely transaction-specific theories are often unequal to the task of capturing a crucial moral dimension which is, again, abundantly developed in structural theories: the responsibility of individual agents to shape social conditions so as to foster human flourishing, and to ensure basic needs and liberties. Structural theories offer us crucial moral insights that are at the heart of what we lament in many exploitative transactions. However, lately, structural concerns have only marginally impacted applied ethicists' and in particular research ethicists' work on exploitation, as the popularity of the economic model testifies. Wertheimer's theory certainly bears part of the blame (Zwolinski 2012; Gray 2020). In my view, there is indeed a huge potential to revive structural accounts of exploitation.

A New Framework for Structural Injustice and Transaction-Specific Exploitation

In the following, let us accept the transaction-specific critique against structuralists. Cases like *Antidote* should be reason enough for this commitment. Nevertheless, I think that many of us feel a strong discomfort when purely transactional theorists, such as Wertheimer (1999, 2011), argue that structural injustice should not be part of a theory of exploitation. To underpin this discomfort, let me start with an intuition that shall direct us toward a new conceptual account that aims to revive structural concerns without animating the transactional critique. *Double Standard Trial* represents real-world incidences of exploitation that appear in repeated patterns and that are characterized by a high degree of "structural prevalence." The existence of structural injustice (including poverty, malnutrition, and lack of access to health care) makes it possible that exploitative health research excessively occurs in LMICs (Malmqvist 2017).

The important question is whether single and isolated events of exploitation, such as *Antidote*, capture all the relevant case features of *Double Standard Trial*. It seems that while structural features are of no concern in the first case, they still matter for the latter one. The intuition here is that any background system—just or unjust—may host isolated cases of exploitation like the one described in *Antidote*, but the exploitation occurring in cases like *Double Standard Trial* is actually reinforced and perpetuated by unjust background conditions. Transaction-specific accounts of exploitation usually conceptualize exploitation in terms of discrete events (i.e., individual transactions). However, I argue that there is a dynamic dimension to exploitation: exploitation can occur as a series of temporally sequenced events or can reoccur in repeated patterns. Here, structural injustice is not the wrong-making feature of any given exploitative event, *per se*, but rather of the persistence or *prevalence* of exploitation as it occurs within the relevant structures.

Accounting for the Prevalence of Exploitation in Unjust Settings: The Conditional Probability Argument

To finally come up with an account for the conceptual connection between background injustice and transaction-specific exploitation, my strategy is to conceptualize the prevalence of exploitation, which seems to be a decisive characteristic of exploitative transactions like *Double Standard Trial*. Such cases repeatedly occur in unjust contexts, precisely because structural injustice makes it easier for exploiters to achieve exploitative deals. The prevalence of exploitation plausibly corresponds to the frequency with which exploitative events occur, given a specified body of transactions, and can subsequently be conceptualized as an event with a certain *expected relative frequency* or *probability of occurrence*.[9]

I argue the following to give credit to the role background injustice plays in determining the prevalence of exploitation: given the universe of possible fair and unfair transactions Ω, let $Z \in \Omega$ be an exploitative transaction and $p(Z)$ its probability of occurrence. It is true for some (but not all) Z that the *conditional probability* of mutually consented and beneficial exploitative transactions Z under unjust background conditions is higher than the probability of mutually consented and beneficial exploitative transactions Z under just background conditions.

$$p(Z|\text{ injustice}) > p(Z|\text{ justice}),$$

where "justice" reflects a structural background with no or only a low level of structural injustice and "injustice" a truly unjust structural background.

The baseline for a minimum number of exploitative events is given by the conditional probability under just background conditions $p(Z|\text{ justice})$. Thus,

I assume that exploitative transactions can happen even in a context of just background structures. I also contend that we can never completely eliminate the occurrence of exploitative transactions, which implies that p(Z) never drops to zero.

The intuition behind the conditional probability argument for structural exploitation is simple. An unjust background is neither necessary nor sufficient for exploitation, but conditions the probability of occurrence of exploitation. This means a conceptual connection between background injustice and exploitation can be established through the relative expected frequency of exploitative events. A single exploitative event may be conceptually independent of background injustice by relations of necessity and sufficiency, but its frequency of occurrence is not, as "injustice" *increases* the conditional probability of unfair transactions Z. Some philosophers have put forward a theory of probabilistic causation underling this "probability raising" relation (Cartwright 1979; Reichenbach 1956; Suppes 1970).[10] Opting for a causal theory seems plausible when variables (here injustice and exploitation) stand in a causal-explanatory relationship. Consider the following example for illustrative purposes:[11]

> *Smoking.* The fact that the conditional probability of lung cancer is increased in smokers does not mean that smoking is either necessary or sufficient for the development of lung cancer. Not every smoker develops lung cancer and not every cancer patient smokes. Nevertheless, there is a probabilistic connection: the probability of developing cancer is higher in smokers. Moreover, there is a causal explanatory connection: we can explain that smoking has caused cancer in a particular patient.[12]

These insights regarding causation, though drawn from an example that cannot strictly be perceived as a normative phenomenon, may be transferable to the case of international health research. More specifically, the analogy is supposed to help conceptualize causation as a link between background injustices and exploitation. In perfectly just contexts, in which regulations, administrative competence, and universal health care protect research subjects from participating in exploitative clinical studies, the risk of exploitation as a structural phenomenon may be negligible. In stark contrast, the probability of exploitation in a LMIC context is often very high: lax regulations, ineffective public administration, and insufficiently developed health care systems enable or *probabilistically cause* exploitative clinical trials. Here, I mean to draw an analogy: just as cancer-causing "factors" contained in cigarette smoke increase the mutation rate of cells, unjust circumstances are "factors" that increase the exploitation rate.[13]

The exploitation rate may even (but does not necessarily) increase over time if structural injustices are not remedied. On the one hand, the "distributive gap" between exploiter and exploited grows over time, as the exploiter gains proportionally more, which makes the exploiter more powerful relative to the exploited. On the other hand, exploitation can become a more easily accepted practice, where exploiters are less willing to adapt to fair rules, as they are not socially or economically sanctioned.

Note that this linear connection between background injustice and the prevalence of exploitation does not necessarily hold. It may be logically possible that a higher frequency of mutually beneficial exploitative events can ameliorate the conditions of the worst off, at least in the long run. To give an example, one may argue that sweatshop labor, even though exploitative, is relatively well paid and can help individuals to get out of absolute poverty (Zwolinski 2012, 161f). This, in turn, may make them less susceptible to being exploited by others.

Systemic and Non-systemic Transactional Exploitation

Based on this analysis, I would like to introduce two subsets of exploitation, that is, *systemic*[14] and *non-systemic* transaction-specific exploitation (Table 6.1). I will define an exploitative event X as a *systemic event* if it shows the following probability pattern: the conditional probability of the exploitative event increases *significantly* under unjust settings, compared to an (negligible) exploitation rate under just circumstances.

Systemic transaction-specific exploitation: $p(X|\text{ injustice}) \gg p(X|\text{ justice})$

where "justice" reflects a structural background with no or only a low level of structural injustice and "injustice" a truly unjust structural background.

The term "systemic" indicates that an exploitative transaction is (mainly) probabilistically caused by unjust background conditions, compared to a counterfactual just world. One striking example of systemic exploitation is *Double Standard Trial*, as the relative expected frequency of exploitative clinical research is certainly significantly higher in unjust contexts. Moreover, the baseline of exploitation in clinical research, the exploitation rate under just circumstances, may not be worth mentioning, as contexts of good regulations, access to health care, and general prosperity rarely allow exploitative trials. As I mentioned before, I do not want to claim that cases of exploitative research can be fully prevented in just societies, but they are at least not pervasive or occurring in systemic patterns.

Next, I will define a "non-systemic" event Y of exploitation as an event with the following probability pattern: the conditional probability of an event Y does *not or only slightly* change(s) under unjust background conditions compared to a just context.

Non-systemic transaction-specific exploitation: $p(Y|\text{ injustice}) \approx p(Y|\text{ justice})$

where "justice" reflects a structural background with no or only a low level of structural injustice and "injustice" a truly unjust structural background.

"Non-systemic" shall indicate that an exploitative transaction is not primarily owed to unjust background conditions and is stochastically (almost) independent of structural factors. Therefore, the exploitation rate of non-systemic exploitation is approximately the same in just and unjust societies, as background injustice does not (significantly) contribute to the occurrence of these cases.[15] The most striking example of non-systemic exploitation may be *Antidote*, where the probability of occurrence of Y is unrelated to the status of background injustice. Note that in *Antidote* the exploiter may be in a weaker social position than the exploited, as we have no information about the structural characteristics of the society they belong to.

Ultimately, the distinction between systemic and non-systemic events of exploitation is an empirical one and needs real-world input. We need to empirically examine whether a specific type of exploitative transaction (*Double Standard Trial*, *Antidote*, etc.) highly or only moderately correlates with background conditions. However, it remains a conceptual undertaking to define when an exploitative practice falls under the category of systemic or non-systemic exploitation. The question is: When, precisely, do we consider exploitation a systemic event whose frequency of occurrence is (significantly)

Table 6.1 Systemic and Non-Systemic Exploitation Compared

	Systemic Exploitation (X)	**Non-Systemic Exploitation (Y)**
Background Conditions: Unjust / Just	$P(X \mid \text{Injustice}) \gg p(X \mid \text{Justice})$	$P(Y \mid \text{Injustice}) \approx p(Y \mid \text{Justice})$
Time	Exploitation rate p(X) at t_1 can **increase** over time, if distributive imbalance or structural injustice between exploiter and exploited increases or if exploitation becomes an accepted practice at t_2. However, exploitation rate p(X) at t_1 can **decrease** if cumulative exploitation leads to a significantly better situation of the exploited at t_2 through the gain of net benefits in exploitative transactions.	Exploitation rate p(Y) is constant over time, exploitation is isolated from other factors, and there is no mutually reinforcing relationship between structural features and exploitation.

increased by background injustice? For instance, emotional exploitation in couples may be a borderline case. While emotional exploitation is surely enhanced by structural discrimination, such as misogyny or gender violence, it is possible that formally just societies with nondiscriminatory and equitable institutions leave room for personal greed, revenge, and malevolence unrelated to structural shortcomings. Here, a more comprehensive account is needed to explain how unjust structures are framed and how they relate to individuals (see, e.g., Young 2009, 2011). Hence, I would like to stipulate that I only aim to capture the difference between the most extreme types of exploitation: cases that clearly have a structural component and cases that are plausibly construed as unrelated to background injustice.

I now anticipate several objections to my framework. First, some may argue that my account of systemic exploitation collapses into the structuralist position. This is mistaken, since I accept the transaction-specific account insofar as I conceptualize systemic exploitation as an agent-relative moral wrong. That is, in an exploitative transaction, the exploiter commits a *prima facie* moral wrong independent of the background conditions. Structural factors are neither sufficient nor necessary to make systemic exploitation wrong. Thus, a single and isolated act of systemic exploitation is pre-structural in the sense that the fairness of a transaction can be evaluated independently of the structural background (see Wertheimer 1999). Unjust structures do not revoke the exploiter's wrongdoing, but make exploitation easier, which is reflected in an augmented exploitation rate for systemic exploitation. I do not believe that the structural position can account for this.

For instance, Roemer (1996) assumes that the unfairness of a transaction hinges on the illegitimacy of the initial asset distribution. Also, both Sample (2003) and Young (2009) advance the view that reflection on structural injustice should lead us to identify as exploitative some actions which, in the absence of injustice, would be considered morally innocent (Wollner 2019; Zwolinski 2012). I disagree; I do not think that structural injustice is the wrong-making feature of exploitative transactions. Rather, background injustice is the wrong-making feature of the systemic persistence of exploitation, measured by its relative expected frequency. In other words, the conceptual connection between background injustice and systemic exploitation concerns the pattern according to which exploitation occurs, not the exploitative act by itself. Further, and also contrary to Roemer, Young, and Sample, I accept that there are other moral "wrong makers" at work in exploitative transactions; these are the factors that make the exploitative act itself illegitimate. Exploitation is more than a symptom of the moral illegitimacy of background structures.

However, my view also accounts for the structuralist intuition that our moral discontent in cases such as *Double Standard Trial* does not only concern the transaction-specific unfairness isolated from background factors; rather, we lament that structural background conditions enable pervasive exploitation, often in the long term. In this regard, concerns articulated in structural theories of exploitation (Cohen 1988, 1989, 1995; Gray 2020; McKeown 2016; Sample 2003, 2018; Wollner 2019; Young 2009) find expression in the concept of systemic exploitation.

This brings me to a second objection, namely, that intermediate transaction-specific theories of exploitation already sufficiently address the dimension of structural injustice. As previously outlined, Malmqvist (2013, 2017) claims that taking advantage of injustice is morally illegitimate, not only because agents who do so wrongfully benefit from the plight of others but also because they maintain and perpetuate structural deficiencies when they exploit. In this regard, the objection contends, the concept of "taking advantage of injustice" adequately captures the structural feature of what I call systemic exploitation. My reply to this is that Malmqvist (2013, 2017) insightfully describes a moral wrong that is deeply connected to systemic exploitation, and which describes the mechanism by which exploiters exert influence on background structures while exploiting in transactions (see Table 6.1). However, Malmqvist's account does not establish a conceptual connection between structural injustice and the prevalence of systemic exploitation, as I do by appeal to probabilistic causation.

I will address this more fully in the Section "Implications of Systemic Exploitation in International Health Research," but it is worth taking a moment now to explain why establishing this conceptual connection is so important. The connection between structural injustice and the prevalence of exploitation has significant consequences for the distribution of responsibilities: if structures are causal factors that bring about exploitation, then responsibility for remediating exploitation is shared between the members of the group responsible for addressing structural injustice and the individual exploiting agent—assuming the exploitative transaction is systemic in character. "Taking advantage of injustice" focuses solely on the moral wrong committed by the exploiter and leaves out the causal contributions of other agents who perpetuate and maintain structural injustice. My account is certainly in line with Malmqvist's, but I am staking out a more far-reaching claim regarding the role of background structures.

Fair Play Model, Structural Injustices, and Community Exploitation

I have argued that standard theories of transactional exploitation inadequately address structural injustices when it comes to systemic cases of exploitation exemplified by *Double Standard Trial.* Since my claim has been that systemic exploitation embodies a concept specific to transactions, I haven't said much about the relationship between structural injustice and *community exploitation*. As I argued when I presented the fair play model, community exploitation is best understood as "free-riding" on the social value produced by a joint enterprise or collaborative effort in health research. The moral wrong committed by researchers and sponsors as well as other stakeholders (including populations in third countries that benefit from a research project) is that some members of a joint enterprise, and most notably research subjects and community members, are afforded an unfairly small part of the benefits at stake in relation to their relative contributions.

However, this is only the ideal part of the fair play model and there is an aspect relevant to non-ideal theory as well: structural injustices considerably hamper the achievement of a fair distribution—regulated by the principle of fair play or stakeholder fairness—among all stakeholders, especially when social and political institutions are defective. The social and political context, the (non)existence of universal health coverage, the general level of infrastructure to supply medicines and so on, are frequently considered to be the major obstacles to fair benefit-sharing in international health research (Buchanan et al. 2011; Holzer 2016; Sonderholm 2010).

This worry is not far-fetched. Ooms et al. (2010) have sustained an argument that relies on the assumption that many LMICs are caught in "poverty traps." Poverty traps are vicious cycles of insufficient capital to build infrastructure, sustain education, build businesses, provide health services, etc.—all the things needed for healthy workers who would produce capital. Poverty traps concern long-term growth and institutional failure and thus constitute a structural problem in poor countries; they are a cause of increasing divergence in the global economy (Azariadis and John 2005). Scholars like Barugahare and Lie (2014) have considered bad governance of poor countries to be another factor that reinforces poverty.

One implication of poverty traps and misconduct in governance concerns access to health care. The World Health Organization (WHO 2025) states that despite the United Nations Sustainable Development Goals, among which is universal health coverage, at least half of the world's population still do not have full coverage of essential health services. As of 2024, extreme poverty remains a significant global challenge. Approximately 8.5 percent of the world's population—about 700 million people—live on less than $2.15 per day, which is the international extreme poverty line. Most of these individuals reside in sub-Saharan Africa and regions affected by conflict or fragility, highlighting the disproportionate burden faced by these areas (World Bank 2025). Severe structural injustice is thus a striking feature of many LMICs and affects people's health capabilities.

While I refrain from defining community exploitation in terms of structural injustice—I will come to this point in a moment—I think that some brief words should be directed toward the implications of structural injustice for community exploitation. The fact that makes structural injustice so important to community exploitation is that the fair value of the knowledge produced in a research project is unlikely to reach the general population of a host community. Due to the magnitude of structural deficits, we probably face this problem in many very poor countries in spite of the presumed goodwill of researchers, sponsors, third countries, and local health authorities.

Structural Exploitation Is Not Community Exploitation

Wenner (2018a) calls for a new framework of community exploitation to leave behind the transactional model and suggests that the "candidate" standing to reason is a *structural* account of exploitation. But does structural exploitation amount to community exploitation? I will restrict my discussion to perhaps the most impactful structural account of exploitation that completely abstracts from exploitative transactions, unlike the accounts suggested by Roemer and Cohen. Iris Young (2009, 70) sustains that the central insight expressed by the concept of exploitation is its manifestation of oppression: it "occurs through a steady process of the transfer of the results of the labor of one social group to benefit another." At first glance, this seems to be in line with my account of community exploitation in the context of health research. Researchers and sponsors, as well as third countries that benefit from health research conducted in LMICs, exploit when they systematically transform host community members' contributions and efforts into their own benefits.

However, Young (2009, 69) aims at a structural account in the sense that she thinks exploitation should go beyond distributive concerns. Exploitation establishes and sustains a "class division that does not consist only in the distributive fact that some people have great wealth while most people have little … Exploitation enacts a structural relation between social groups." These relations are produced and reproduced through a structural process that eventually maintains and augments the power, status, and wealth of the advantaged (Young 2011, 14).

What does Young (2009) mean when she says that "exploitation enacts structural relations between social groups"? Her account appears to suggest that something like a relational structure emerges from the interaction of different groups (Young 2011, Ch. 5). In particular, I suspect that Young's basic structure would entail a "thick" relational account among those different groups, which would, in turn, suggest a need for principles of justice to regulate these interactions. This would be tantamount to the "basic structure model" defended by Wenner (2018a). Again, there are many other frameworks that advocate a much broader definition of "structure," which includes agents acting in a global context (Beitz 1979; Pogge 2002).

Having argued against the claim that a research enterprise is best understood as a basic structure (Chapter 4), I contend that it is equally mistaken to frame community exploitation as a form of structural exploitation. Beyond that, my reasoning comes down to the concern transactional theorists raise: there are exploitative events that are unrelated to structural injustice, and there are fair transactions taking place in a context of structural injustice. Structures are neither necessary nor sufficient to make exploitation occur. Similarly, a single event of community exploitation is independent of structural concerns. Communities, understood as legitimate stakeholders in a joint research enterprise, can be afforded fair benefits in the context of an individual clinical trial despite a global macro process of "structural exploitation" in which a financial elite uses the results of the labor of the global poor to benefit themselves (see Young 2011). Vice versa, communities can be exploited in relatively just contexts, demonstrated by so-called "me-too drug trials" – which, recall, are studies that test a drug similar to already approved treatments, whose development has no potential to generate an additional benefit to future patients (Wendler and Rid 2017, 80; Ch. 5). These trials frequently take place in HICs, i.e., in relatively just contexts where sponsoring companies want to increase their profits.

In consequence, structural injustices are neither necessary nor sufficient for community exploitation. Instead of making structures the conceptual and justificatory underpinning of exploitation, I think that structures find expression in another moral concern, further downstream in the argument. Structures, and more specifically structural injustices, are (non-ideal) obstacles to the (ideal) realization of fair research according to the principle of fairness. My account thus constitutes a categorical difference from those of the structuralists, such as Young (2009, 2011), McKeown (2016), Wollner (2019) or Gray (2020), who define exploitation as a form of structural phenomenon. Such structuralists argue that structural processes producing vulnerabilities to deprivation and domination as well as the systematic perpetuation of these structural injustices together build the moral content of exploitation. In contrast, I contend that community exploitation is simply distributive injustice within a cooperative scheme with a joint end. Structural injustice is then a hindrance when we want to achieve fair benefit-sharing, but it is not the moral content of community exploitation.

A Framework for Structures and Community Exploitation

In the previous section I argued that structural concerns impact community exploitation insofar as the socially valuable benefits of research are mostly bestowed on more powerful agents. As a short digression, I would like to deepen our understanding of how this can be the case.

The structural defects of a system are usually accepted and acknowledged self-reinforcing patterns. Wiedenbrug (2018) distinguishes two types of vicious cycles that imprint themselves onto structural processes: "structural-relational" and "structural-systemic" contributions to injustice. Structural-relational contributions are the contributions of individual agents to the production and reproduction of structural injustice, which can be individuated (Wiedenbrug 2018, 96). In this case, an agent can be identified who enables the structures to make exploitation more likely. Malmqvist (2017) appeals to a structural-relational account when he introduces the moral wrong of "taking advantage of injustice." Researchers and sponsors and other "accomplices" can be identified as agents that intentionally take advantage of background injustices when they conduct "cheap trials." "Cheap trials" do not only refer to trials under a double standard that primarily exploit research subjects, but also to trials with a low social value and/or where an unfairly small part of the social value accrues to a host community.

Structural-systemic contributions to injustice, on the other hand, go beyond individual agents' responsibilities and concern the whole "game" that is played. This is what Young (2011, 52) calls "structural injustice." According to Young (2011, 52), structural injustice is morally problematic, but distinct from the wrongful actions of individual agents, or even the repressive policies of a state. Structural injustice emerges from the consequences of many individuals and institutions pursuing their individual interests, within the limits of accepted rules and norms.

On the structural-systemic level, all participants in the "game" and its rules have a position of advantage or disadvantage. Differently put, we all conform to the system in which we act and live, and in this way we contribute to the maintenance of the very same system. This concerns both the options agents have within the system and the internalization of the rules and the logic of our structures. The structural-systemic phenomenon occurs in the global research system, dominated by few global players in the pharmaceutical industry and governmental researchers and sponsors mostly from HICs. It seems many low-income countries suffer from a chronic capital insufficiency and underdeveloped infrastructure (Ooms et al. 2010). Since they are unable to develop their own research systems, they depend on foreign researchers and sponsors. Furthermore, the rules of how research is done, and this includes, e.g., a patent-based regime under the TRIPS agreement, are patterns on a global level. Structural injustices in the research system thus find themselves reinforced by the agents that align with these rules.

In this regard, I contend that structural injustices matter. They complement the fair play model and allow a full-fledged depiction of moral concerns in the debate on the fair distribution of benefits. Both structural-relational and structural-systemic contributions to structural injustice have a significant impact on the frequency with which community exploitation occurs. The probabilistic argument for transaction-specific exploitation similarly applies to community exploitation. Background injustice is the wrong-making feature of the systemic persistence (maintained through structural-relational or structural-systemic patterns) of community exploitation, measured by the exploitation rate. The conceptual connection between background injustice and community exploitation concerns the pattern in which exploitative clinical trials occur, not community exploitation itself. In this sense, my previous conclusions for systemic transactional exploitation from the Section "A New Framework for Structural Injustice and Transaction-Specific Exploitation" are transferrable to a nontransactional account of community exploitation grounded in fairness obligations *across cooperative schemes*. While the fair play model still plays the leading role of setting a fairness norm in a cooperative research enterprise, structural injustices indicate whether an ideal fair outcome can be (easily) achieved given the circumstances.

To summarize, community exploitation is systemic, not structural. I will not outline the argument in its entirety, but it will be helpful to say the following: I argued that community exploitation can be framed as a moral wrong committed by some stakeholders of a cooperative scheme, such as a research enterprise, when they free-ride on the efforts of other stakeholders, that is, when they do not return a fair share to those who have similarly submitted to cooperation. Now, the exploitation rate of exploitative trials, in terms of community exploitation, is significantly higher in contexts of the structural injustice usually prevalent in LMICs. I therefore assume that the overall exploitation rate of unfair trials in LMICs is higher than in HICs.[16] For that reason, it is advisable to complement my account of community exploitation with a conceptual account including background injustices and with the demand that the background conditions in host communities be improved (see next Section "Implications of Systemic Exploitation in International Health Research"). This would eventually make fair benefits for host communities a more likely outcome of research.

Implications of Systemic Exploitation in International Health Research

In this section, I will discuss the implications from my previous account, especially for the case of systemic exploitation in international health research. The implications are related to the importance of background injustice within a theory of exploitation, the moral responsibilities of different agents to prevent exploitation and to remedy background injustice, as well as the legal permissibility of exploitative research trials.

The Importance of Structural Injustice within a Theory of Exploitation

We may have good reasons to direct our attention to structural injustice following the original concern by Cohen and Roemer, at least as far as systemic incidences of exploitation are concerned. We can push that intuition even further and argue that our normative focus ought to be the remediation of structural injustice to prevent both systemic transaction-specific and systemic community exploitation in the first place. Even though structural injustice does not necessarily lead to exploitation (and is not sufficient to explain it), the prevalence of structural injustice is probabilistically related to the prevalence of systemic exploitation through its probability-increasing property. In other words, background injustice gains normative significance through its connection to the systemic persistence of exploitation. Much like I argued in Section "A New Framework for Structural Injustice and Transaction-Specific Exploitation," I argue here that we can capture this intuition by referring to the smoking analogy.

> *Anti-Smoking Campaigns.* It is reasonable to argue that smoking increases the conditional probability of cancer. Then, it seems to be normatively appropriate to vindicate anti-smoking campaigns that aim to prevent cancer genesis and to save lives. This, however, does not entail that preventive measures would eventually lead to a complete eradication of cancer. We still have good reasons to spend health resources on research into and development of cancer treatments that directly target the disease.

Analogous to anti-smoking campaigns, the remediation of structural injustice ought to be one major focus if our goal is to prevent systemic exploitation.[17] Without a stable unjust structure that permits systemic exploitation, exploitation cannot prevail, at least not as a systemic practice. However, taking up the analogy of cancer treatment, we should not lose sight of the moral wrong of either transaction-specific or community exploitation itself: we ought to remedy and morally condemn exploitation despite the importance of structural factors.

Unlike structuralists, I do not think that "structures" bear moral liability and responsibility for the wrongs done through exploitative transactions. Individual agents are morally responsible and liable for their acts of mutually advantageous transaction-specific exploitation. Differently put, unjust structures only create the "right" circumstances for exploiters to wrong others and thus make exploitation easier, but they are not determinative of exploitative transactions.

My impression is that both structuralists and transactional theorists advocate extreme and perhaps implausible positions: while the former places weight exclusively on the unjust system as the determinative factor in exploitation, the latter underemphasizes the responsibilities of other very important agents that in some way also restrict the action space of the exploiter and the exploited. As mentioned above, I share the point with transactional theorists that the exploiter as a free and autonomous agent is at the end the primarily responsible and liable person, *if* it is finally (which I assume to be the case) in her power to take unfair advantage of another person or not.

Furthermore, an issue related to this discussion is that the distinction between systemic and non-systemic exploitation points to a recurrent critique in moral philosophy, namely, that ignoring real-world factors in abstract case examples frequently leads to wrong conclusions relative to a particular context (see Wilson 2009; Wolff 1998). Indeed, what I call non-systemic incidences of exploitation mostly refer to abstract thought experiments, such as *Antidote*, that often resemble unlikely and hypothetical events brought up by moral philosophers to defend the consistency of certain moral concepts (see Wolff 1998). But do the conclusions from *Antidote* hold for real-world contexts, such as clinical research? In defense of abstract examples, we may concede that they are necessary to point to the underlying moral arguments and concerns that are of conceptual interest. Regarding exploitation, purely transactional theorists use abstract examples to point out that structural injustice should not be our primary moral concern when it comes to exploitation. Rather, the salient moral wrong of exploitation is that an individual party takes unfair advantage of another party.

Then, I think that the introduction of systemic, as opposed to non-systemic, exploitation makes sense, precisely when it comes to the moral weight of background injustice in relation to exploitative transactions and/or community exploitation. The concept of systemic exploitation reintroduces the specifics[18] of more "realistic" cases of exploitation that prevail within and due to unjust contexts. Hence, unjust structures have much greater moral significance for systemic exploitation than non-systemic exploitation. It seems that the distinction between systemic and non-systemic exploitation helps us understand that there can be different moral concerns—structural injustice, but also personal motives, interpersonal wrongdoing, or a lack of compliance with the rules of fair play—in exploitative acts, which are sometimes more and sometimes less normatively salient. This is missing in the transactional and particularly in the economic model.

Finally, it seems to me that abstract examples related to non-systemic exploitation have undermined the importance of background injustice and overemphasized individual wrongdoing in cases of systemic exploitation, which is the type of exploitation we are worried about in clinical research. This may revive concerns by structuralists that (systemic) exploitation induces moral discomfort precisely because the structural background enables more powerful agents to exploit the vulnerable.

Moral Responsibilities to Remedy Background Injustices

My point in the section "The Importance of Structural Injustice within a Theory of Exploitation" yields a direct impact for the moral responsibilities that agents bear to remedy background injustice with the final aim of preventing exploitation. Purely transaction-specific accounts, and most notably the economic model, implicitly assume that the exploiter—in this case mainly researchers and sponsors—is the only party morally responsible for preventing and remedying exploitation. Consequently, they seek remedies inside the transaction, such as more benefits for the exploited party, fairer compensation, etcetera (see Emanuel et al. 2008). In contrast, the structural account extends the realm of moral responsibilities to agents other than the exploiter, that is, to all agents that are responsible for remedying structural injustice. The intuition drawn from structuralists suggests that the prevention of exploitation first and foremost happens through the remediation of background injustice. I think this structural intuition has great potential to inform our moral assessment of systemic exploitation. Fixing structural injustice should eventually be reflected in a reduced rate of systemic exploitation.

Hence, taking structures as causal factors seriously means that responsibility for exploitation is broadly held: it is certainly held by the exploiter, but also held in part by other agents, who stand outside the exploitative transaction. Sometimes, structures are not causally implicated in exploitation, such as in cases of non-systemic exploitation. However, when it comes to systemic exploitation, as represented by *Double Standard Trial*, those who help restrict the action possibilities of exploiters and those who exploit bear responsibilities, as they consolidate the pattern (or rate) with which exploitative transactions occur.

But who are these responsible agents? Young (2011, 143) draws a distinction between the concepts of *responsibility* and *duty* (the second of which is also synonymously used with obligation). Unlike duties, responsibilities are more open-ended, meaning there is no specification of what actions they require. Furthermore, responsibilities are less obligatory than perfect duties. Taking responsibility allows greater exercise of discretion than enacting a duty does. I refrain from deepening any account of responsibility,[19] as this would go beyond the scope of this book, which focuses on obligations. However, let me briefly outline some thoughts on this matter. I do not pretend to offer a full catalog of agents that may be responsible for remedying background injustices. Rather, I provide some ideas about who these agents could be in the context of health research.

The most dominant normative model for attributing responsibilities to agents in the literature is grounded in the liability of actors. An agent can be held liable and thus responsible when it is possible to establish a causal link between her action and the outcome. This "liability model of responsibility" is "backward-looking" in the sense that responsibility is assigned for an act that occurred in the past (Wiedenbrug 2018, 150).

Opposed to the liability model, Young (2011, Ch. 3) proposes a "forward-looking" model for the attribution of responsibilities—the "social connection model." Young's (2011) account holds that all agents who contribute to a structural process that results in injustice are held responsible. It is "forward-looking" in the sense that all agents ought to take collective action to change the unjust structures. Individual responsibilities arise in relation to issues of structural injustice and all of us who are implicated in unjust structural processes bear responsibilities. Young (2011, Ch. 3) here relies on Arendt's (1987) distinction between *guilt*—individual agents are guilty in the sense that they are liable for their misdeeds—and *collective responsibility*, where people belonging to a system collectively bear responsibilities to change corrupt and unjust systems. Young (2011, Chapter 5) holds that the scope of the social connection model is global. It cannot be based on membership in a group or nation because we participate directly in the operations of (global) institutions that together produce injustice.

Transferring these insights to offshored clinical research, it certainly seems justified to attribute responsibilities under the liability model to individual actors that have primarily contributed to the unjust structures the citizens of a host country suffer within. Of course, holding these actors responsible presupposes that they have a certain action space and are not completely constrained by the "rules of the game" or some super-structure. Frequently, representatives of national governments, research ethics committees, and health authorities can and should be held liable to improve local health care and research systems so as to make host communities less susceptible to accepting or hosting exploitative clinical trials (Barugahare 2016; Wenner 2016). Solely blaming the sponsoring agencies leaves out the moral responsibilities of agents that have contributed to a structural environment that fosters and maintains systemic exploitation.

Looking through the lens of the social connection model, responsibilities can be considerably expanded. Individual actors, including representatives and members of HICs and also LMICs, and international institutions collectively maintain and even reinforce injustices. For instance, Pogge (2008) has previously criticized the international patent system under the TRIPS agreement on the grounds that it hugely disfavors research on drugs to alleviate the disease burden in LMICs (Holzer and Pogge 2020). Governments in affluent countries bear responsibilities for the structural conditions in which drugs are tested and provided to citizens through national health services. Given that all of us participate in globalized systems, every one of us bears responsibilities to contribute to structural reforms wherever possible in order to remove structural injustices that exist on a large scale. This is even true for research subjects in LMICs: they might bear to a certain extent responsibilities to forgo participation in exploitative research to signal to other actors that the current practice needs to be changed (Rivera Lopez 2017, 19).

The Permissibility of Exploitation

The revival of structural concerns in the context of systemic exploitation may have implications for the legal permissibility of exploitation. Here, I will just sketch some possible lines of argument without attempting to be comprehensive. However, I will deepen the discussion in Chapter 8.[20]

Many have objected to the fact that offshored clinical research associated with exploitative research designs is still permitted (Mitra 2012; Wenner 2016). However, Wertheimer (1999, 289–93, 2011) has previously challenged the demand to ban exploitative research from the international domain on grounds of the "non-worseness claim." In short, the non-worseness claim states that an interaction between A and B cannot be morally worse than no interaction at all if A and B are both better off compared to a baseline of no interaction (Malmqvist 2017, 478). This is the case in *Double Standard Trial*, as the exploited party B gains a net benefit through her participation. In the same vein, we can argue that communities are better off when they host exploitative research than when they forgo the possibility. This does not imply that it is morally permissible for A, the exploiter, to exploit. Rather, Wertheimer means to say that it is wrong for third parties (like regulatory agencies, governments, or research ethics committees) to prevent Pareto superior win-win transactions on the ground that such transactions are unfair (Wertheimer 2011, 256ff). Note that Wertheimer's argument is based on the assumption that the prohibition of exploitative research would give researchers and sponsors a reason to forgo mutually beneficial trials in LMICs. In a different argument (the "strategic argument"), Wertheimer (2008, 81) says that the prohibition of exploitation can be legitimate, but only if it incentivizes parties to transact fairly.

I have two thoughts about this. First, several authors have challenged the non-worseness claim. As I have explained, Malmqvist (2013, 2017) offers a structural argument based on the moral wrong of taking advantage of injustice, which is unrelated to the moral wrong of exploitation, but which may set a constraint on the permissibility of exploitation. Exploiters, such as pharmaceutical companies, take advantage of injustice and maintain the unjust conditions that have enabled exploitation. This can eventually serve as a moral foundation for prohibiting exploitative interactions despite the fact that this would lead to Pareto inferior outcomes in the short run.[21] My account of systemic exploitation may follow this argumentative line. We may argue that systemic exploitation should be banned because exploitative practices themselves foster and enable unjust background conditions, as researchers and sponsors take advantage of prevalent injustices without remediating them, and simultaneously contribute to the notion that the agents primarily responsible for background injustice (e.g., the governments of host countries) are not morally required to remediate them. Reinforced background injustices, in turn, make systemic exploitation itself more likely. Following this argument, the prohibition of exploitative research stands to reason: banning exploitation would contribute to the remediation of background injustices in the long run, which reduces the exploitation rate. Yet, we should not forget that this comes along with costs for research subjects and communities in the short run, as potential benefits are forgone.

Second, the argument just presented might not hold in the long run. As I tried to clarify in Section "A New Framework for Structural Injustice and Transaction-Specific Exploitation," a linear connection between systemic exploitation and background injustice does not necessarily exist in the long run. The fact that exploited parties gain absolutely, even though not relatively, from exploitative transactions, may lead to fewer exploitative transactions. As I argued, this seems to a certain extent plausible, for instance, for people who live in absolute poverty and who can be helped through exploitative labor (see

Zwolinksi 2012). Eventually, extremely poor people may be able to ascend from absolute poverty to a "minimally decent life," which renders them less susceptible to future exploitation.

This argument rests on the assumption that mutually beneficial exploitation can lead to the mitigation of severe structural injustice. However, I am not convinced that this argument can be made applicable to offshored health research. Here, structural conditions seem to be very complex and have a greater direct impact on the vulnerability of potential research subjects and community members. Even if research subjects and communities gain from an experimental trial, it often seems that the benefits they receive do not ameliorate their health situation in the long run, especially when post-trial access to drugs and reasonable availability and accessibility of care are not guaranteed. Structural changes would need to be of more significant nature, given the current context, to place research subjects and community members in a situation in which they would be considerably less prone to exploitative research.

Concluding Remarks

This chapter proceeded from a moral complaint many authors have when it comes to the charge of exploitation in the context of offshored clinical research: framing exploitation in purely transaction-specific terms leaves out the structural factors that primarily lead to exploitation. To account for this, I addressed the charge of exploitation from a transactional and structural point of view and offered a novel conceptual link between systemic transaction-specific exploitation and structural injustice by adhering to the conditional probability argument. In a second step, I aimed to show that the very same argument holds for community exploitation: we can link structural injustices and the occurrence of community exploitation using the conditional probability argument. As a result of my inquiry, I argued that *systemic exploitation* is the category we need to focus on when referring to exploitative research trials.

Eventually, I showed that structural features or the context in which research is conducted impact the success of fair benefit-sharing. An account of systemic exploitation can consequently *complement* the fair play model as to render it sensitive to the moral status of the background context. The remediation of background injustice positively supports a host community's capacity to take effective advantage of fair benefits according to the principle of fairness, which is internal to a cooperative scheme. This eventually yields normative implications regarding the importance of structural concerns for a theory of community exploitation, moral responsibilities to remedy background injustices, and the permissibility of exploitation in offshored health research.

7

Principles, Procedures, and Mechanisms for Safeguarding Fair Benefits: Reply to Fundamental Objection (iii)

Making Benefits Tangible

After having dedicated the past chapters to the justification requirement, with the aim of grounding the fair play model, let us now have a look at the content requirement. I still owe the reader a specification of when and under what conditions host communities are treated on fair terms (i.e., are not exploited). The content requirement addresses not only the type or substance of benefits but also possible principles and procedures of distributive justice that provide criteria for evaluating whether an attained distribution of benefits is just. There is a vast literature on principles and procedures relevant to distributive justice, traditionally based on the distribution of income, wealth, opportunities, jobs, welfare, utility, and other goods. The Anglo-American literature has highlighted in past decades principles related to egalitarian distributive justice, including Rawls' (TJ, TJR) principle of fair equality of opportunity as well as his difference principle.[1] Principles based on welfare or desert have also been well-represented; so have libertarian principles and frameworks for procedural fairness (Elster 1992, chap. 2; Lamont 2017a).[2]

I have criticized the economic model for providing an insufficiently developed account of how fair benefits might be safeguarded (Chapter 3). I noted that a procedural requirement (in the form of free and noncoerced negotiations) that allows benefits to be traded off between host communities and researchers and sponsors can easily lead to unfair outcomes. Negotiations, even under relatively fair circumstances (e.g., when transparent access to information about the market is guaranteed), can convert research into an auction block. This means that outcomes do not correspond to the fair price that is hypothetically achieved on an ideal market (London and Zollman 2010).[3]

Since the vulnerability model restricts the content of benefits to trials that test drugs or other medical interventions with the aim of addressing health needs and making the intervention available to communities, it seems, at first glance, that benefits are sufficiently specified and guaranteed. However, the vulnerability model lacks a justification for its content specification (Chapter 3) and, moreover, may be too restrictive regarding fair benefits. This is of special importance if we think that cooperative ventures produce valuable informational and noninformational benefits in addition to the tested intervention.

The two main aims of this chapter will oppose both the economic model and the vulnerability model in the following way: the first aim is to offer an account for the content of "fair benefits" in international health research. Benefits under the fair play model are tied to the production of socially valuable knowledge in the strict sense and to the cooperative enterprise of research in the broad sense. This account neither allows for trading off benefits that are completely unrelated to the primary aim of a research study nor restricts fair benefits to the content requirements of responsiveness to health needs and availability alone. As a second aim, I would like to evaluate two alternatives to *fair negotiations*, the main procedural principle for safeguarding benefits in the economic model, as well as alternative mechanisms for fair benefit-sharing. To state it upfront, my inquiry does *not* appeal to a systematic review of the content of fair benefits, distributive principles, procedures, and adequate mechanisms to safeguard benefits. I rather outline some common ideas and concepts present in the research ethics literature. A systematic review would go beyond the scope of this book. Here, I solely aim to present a proof of concept of the fair play model, that is, how fair play can be applied more concretely to questions down-stream of the ethical justification for fair benefit-sharing.

For this purpose, the chapter will be divided into the following sections: I will outline and evaluate the possible content of fair benefits in Section "Fair Benefits under the Fair Play Model," considering the current literature on fair benefits in light of the fair play model. Section "Distributive Principles and Procedures" will focus on a distributive principle and a procedural framework that have both been discussed in the context of justice in health. Angela Ballantyne (2010a) advocates the maximin rule and an adaptation of Rawls' (TJ, TJR) difference principle to health research. Norman Daniels (1996, 2008) and James Sabin (Daniels and Sabin 2002) propose a framework of procedural fairness, or what is commonly known as "accountability for reasonableness." This is actually a key reference for resource allocation in health care, which, I argue, could also be of great utility in assessing the case of international health research. I will further contend that fair benefit-sharing should be institutionalized in the long run to safeguard fair benefits and just benefit-sharing procedures. Section "Mechanisms" then addresses possible institutional mechanisms aimed at guaranteeing fair benefits. This is further downstream from the problem of attaining an adequate distributive principle or fair procedures. Here, I selectively focus on some of the most original and most widely discussed proposals, namely, a global research tax, a reformed global patent regime, prior research agreements, community engagement, and mechanisms to enhance transparency.[4]

Fair Benefits under the Fair Play Model

Current research guidelines and general ethics codes require that benefits from scientific research activity should be shared, with particular attention to the needs of LMICs (UNESCO 2005, articles 2(f) and 15). However, the literature has no univocal answer to the question of what kind of benefits should be shared. As stated in previous chapters, the CIOMS-WHO guidelines (2016, guideline 1) address this by making the social value the ultimate purpose of any research project, where the produced knowledge must be significant to health problems and ought to contribute to the creation or evaluation of interventions, policies, and practices that promote individual and public health. The Declaration of Helsinki (WMA 2013, paragraph 20) specifies, stating one of the two requirements formulated by the vulnerability model, that research must address the health needs and priorities of a community.

To bring clarity, let me review the essential features of the fair play model: obligations of benefit-sharing are created by research conducted as a joint enterprise with the end of generating some instrumental epistemic value that can be obtained from the knowledge gained, manifested in either potential health improvements of a representative cross-section of community members or improvements to public health and/or research-related infrastructure (Chapter 4). If research does not generate information that can be used for these purposes, then research does not constitute a valuable or justifiable enterprise despite other potential benefits associated with it. The intuition is that everyone—researchers, sponsors, other affluent agents, research subjects, and members of host communities—jointly contributes to a medical progress system from which everyone ideally benefits (London and Kimmelman 2008; Mitra 2012).

The fair play model thus follows in particular the current CIOMS-WHO guidelines (2016), as benefits under fair play are subject to fairness considerations associated with the social value of research. In this regard, we can *ex ante* hold that benefits to communities include access to the generated scientific and technological knowledge as well as the provision of new diagnostic or therapeutic modalities or products stemming from it, i.e., the "translated" social knowledge. Moreover, benefits associated with a research enterprise in a broader sense comprise support for health services related to the provision of the tested intervention, i.e., capacity building and infrastructural improvements for research purposes together with the necessary upkeep of technologies, and other benefits associated with the production of socially valuable knowledge.

The fair play model presents an alternative to both the economic model and the vulnerability model. While the economic model leaves the kind of benefits that can be negotiated open, the vulnerability model envisions a narrow conception of what fair benefits potentially are, namely, the post-trial availability of a tested intervention (assuming it is proven successful) that is relevant to local health needs. In the following, I will discuss how exactly the fair play model makes a compromise between the two extremes (these being no limitations to benefits and too-strict limitations). Benefits related to the social value of knowledge (strict interpretation of fair play) and research as a cooperative enterprise (broad interpretation of fair play) are perhaps a middle way, which takes into account the value that can be added to health and health systems through research more generally.

Possible Benefits and Their Evaluation under the Fair Play Model

After having conducted interviews with sixty-nine investigators, senior study staff, and field coordinators doing public health research in South Asia (Bangladesh, Nepal and India), Holly Taylor and Maria Merritt (2011, 1) outline what kind of benefits investigators provided to host communities as well as their self-reported reasons for providing such benefits. According to the authors, community-wide benefits were directed to the health and well-being of the population. The most common types of benefits delivered were the facilitation of access to health care and emergency response to natural disasters. Additionally, other benefits were listed, such as the provision of preventive interventions to community members, delivery of basic health messages, support for public health campaigns, and access to specialty services (Merritt 2011, 3).

Goeffrey Lairumbi et al. (2012) conducted a series of interviews in Kenya, where participants were drawn from within the broader health research system in Kenya. They included researchers from the mainstream health research institutions, teaching hospital staff, policymakers, institutional review board members, representatives of civil society organizations, and community representatives. According to these interviewees, international health research should provide benefits that address both micro- and macro-level issues of justice. In particular, benefits should include access to investigational products and care, training of health personal, what the authors call "brain gain" or "capacity strengthening," and infrastructure improvements, such as technology transfer, expansion of bed capacities, provision of ambulances, and technical training for local health care workers. Furthermore, benefits may consist in supporting community mobilization for health-seeking behaviors, the provision of social amenities, e.g., school fees or plows for farming. Last, benefits may include medical products and public health tools (Lairumbi et al. 2012, 3f).

Dorcas M. Kamuya et al. (2014) conducted another study in Kenya on benefit negotiation and issues related to benefits in practice. Findings reported relate to a social science study in 2010 that explored interactions between fieldworkers and participants in two community-based studies on the Kenyan Coast and more precisely at the KEMRI-Wellcome Trust Research Programme, a biomedical research center established in 1989. According to the authors, wider community benefits were associated with the improvement of local health services through provision of (essential) drugs and additional clinical staff; water treatment for all communal water points; and provision of medical aid during a cholera epidemic including drugs, staff, and referrals. Furthermore, buildings were renovated and equipment provided (Kamuya et al. 2014, 6). Kamuya et al.'s (2014) study also reports that provision of study benefits appeared to be a significant challenge for researchers and fieldworkers, as some participants requested benefits such as food, school fees and uniforms, and shelter.[5] This was beyond what the study team and the research program could provide (Kamuya et al. 2014, 11). Of course, these earlier studies should be contextualized within the current critique of global health research and policy practices, which continue to reflect patterns established during the colonial era, including unequal power dynamics between HICs and LMICs. As many authors argue, there are patterns in who sets research priorities, who controls funding, and whose knowledge is valued. Decolonization would require not only discussing what constitutes fair benefits but also restructuring these relationships to ensure equitable decision-making, local leadership, and the inclusion of diverse perspectives, so that also historically and globally marginalized communities have meaningful influence over health research and policies that affect them (Kwete et al. 2022; Amri et al. 2025; Amri et al. 2025). Although this debate goes beyond the scope of this book, I aim to address its core by discussing mechanisms for implementing fair benefits, particularly through "community engagement" (Section "Community Engagement"), which seek to address power imbalances and ensure decision-making by the communities involved.

However, to limit the debate for now to the content of benefits, it is useful to synthesize the empirical findings from Taylor and Merritt (2011), Lairumbi et al. (2012), and Kamuya et al. (2014). I will organize both realized and aspirational benefits into distinct categories. The interviews describe benefits associated with (i) access to and post-trial availability of the tested intervention, (ii) access to the created knowledge, (iii) access to health care unrelated to research, (iv) the fostering of public health unrelated to research, (v) humanitarian aid, (vi) capacity building, (vii) infrastructural improvements related to the generation of knowledge, (viii) infrastructural improvements unrelated to research, and, last, (xi) other social benefits (see Table 7.1). I argue that obligations of fair benefit-sharing under the fair play model can include (i), (ii), (vi), and (vii), but not (iii), (iv), (v), (viii), and (xi).

The rationale is simple: obligations of fair benefit-sharing only concern research as a joint enterprise among researchers, sponsors, host communities, and other stakeholders (such as countries and their citizens who make use of the produced knowledge). This is related to the view that social value is the primary purpose of any clinical trial and that research should be understood as a collaborative scheme. In this regard, potential benefits under the fair play model comprise the created data or knowledge of a drug, medical intervention, or technology under investigation; the post-trial availability of "translational" benefits of the knowledge, i.e., the drug or technology once proven effective; and the research procedure necessary for drug testing and for related public health improvements.

Nevertheless, other benefits associated with and created through a research enterprise as an activity in the broader sense may equally help sustain and develop local health and health systems of community members. Capacity-strengthening and infrastructure improvements *tied to* a joint enterprise can equally be considered fair benefits created by the stakeholders that participate in a joint cooperative scheme. However, we may say that these benefits resulting from the mere activity are secondary and cannot be justified on their own if the justification of the research—to create socially valuable knowledge—is lacking. Secondary benefits can count as cooperative benefits, but do not replace the demand that some primary benefits, related to socially valuable knowledge, must accrue to communities.

Other benefits beyond research as a cooperative venture, such as the provision of health care unrelated to the joint enterprise, infrastructure like the improvement of schools, the provision of humanitarian aid, and the conduct of public health campaigns, cannot be demanded from researchers and sponsors, at least not under the assumption that researchers and sponsors ought to provide such benefits because they bear special obligations. Rather, what is asked from cooperating agents is that they owe a fair share of the research benefits to those who have contributed to creating them. This, however, does not preclude the claim that researchers, sponsors, and HICs bear another duty of beneficence or even rescue that can be discharged by offering benefits unrelated to research as a joint enterprise. The fair play model leaves it to the researchers and sponsors to decide on whether they provide other benefits.

It seems useful to clarify two points. First, since the provision of benefits unrelated to research does not fall under obligations of benefit-sharing, such provision is better understood as compliance with a (different) duty of beneficence. These other benefits cannot be traded off with the ones related to the generation of socially valuable knowledge in view of the main justification and intention of research as a joint activity. Importantly, a research enterprise and thus the distribution of benefits and burdens *resulting from research cooperation* must be fair in itself. Differently put, the fair play model demands that enough socially valuable benefits resulting from drug or intervention testing accrue to communities.

Second, there may be some class of necessary investments associated with research that are declared to be benefits to communities, for instance, the modernization of research facilities. The fair play model is generous with these kinds of secondary benefits. It is nevertheless important to note that secondary benefits ought to be sustainable: they should show some instrumental value for the improvement of health or the health and research system in the respective host community. For instance, the modernization of technology for a research enterprise can only count as a valuable benefit if the technology is used to further the local health or research system regarding future projects or if the technology is sustainably used, which usually requires training of health personnel that furthermore keep the technology in good condition. This line of reasoning is, for instance, specified in the "Continued Access to Investigational Medicines Guidance Document" published by the Multi-Regional Clinical Trial Center (MRCT) Harvard: a continued access plan in research should include equipment, maintenance, and the training required to maintain the equipment (MRCT 2017, 47). If this is not guaranteed, the modernization of technology (or infrastructure) needed to produce socially valuable knowledge counts as a necessary burden on researchers and sponsors but cannot be considered an appropriate benefit for host communities.

Three Normative Models for Fair Benefits: A Comparison

The vulnerability model considers appropriate all benefits associated with investigated medicines, technologies, and other medical interventions as long as the research question of a trial is responsive to local health needs and goes along with the aim to assure post-trial availability of the corresponding knowledge and interventions (Glantz et al. 1998).[6] At first glance, it seems that the strategy of the fair play model resembles to a great extent the vulnerability model: there are content requirements that limit the scope of fair benefits. However, the fair play model not only allows access to the tested intervention and/or knowledge but also benefits that are related to the accomplishment of a research enterprise, including capacity-building and infrastructure improvements that potentially lead to long-lasting health benefits for community members (see Table 7.1). We should nevertheless emphasize that one central concern of the fair play model is that the tested intervention and the corresponding knowledge be made available to the communities. Of course, every research trial must be carefully evaluated. It may be enough to provide capacity-building related to the knowledge creation and infrastructural improvements if this is a core concern of the research question.

In contrast to the fair play and the vulnerability models, the economic model does not set limits on the content of fair benefits: there is no "main" benefit at stake, such as socially valuable research knowledge, from which every party ought to benefit fairly. This is, however, in conflict with the primary justification of research: research is only justified if it generates socially valuable knowledge. Even Emanuel himself (Emanuel et al. 2000, 2004), the main defender of the economic model, advocates this position in previous works. Another problem is that the economic model is based on the belief that community representatives freely negotiate benefits of "true value" for community members. However, this may not always be the case, especially

Table 7.1 Comparison of the Three Ethical Models Regarding the (Required and/or Permissible) Content of Fair Benefits

	Vulnerability model	Economic model	Fair play model
(i) Access to and post-trial availability of the tested intervention	Yes (if responsive to health needs and/or priorities)	Yes	Yes
(ii) Access to the created knowledge	Yes (only if necessary to address health needs and/or priorities)	Yes	Yes
(iii) Access to health care unrelated to research	No*	Yes	No*
(iv) Fostering of public health unrelated to research	No*	Yes	No*
(v) Humanitarian aid	No*	Yes	No*
(vi) Capacity-building	No*	Yes	Yes
(vii) Infrastructural improvements related to research	No*	Yes	Yes
(viii) Infrastructural improvements unrelated to research	No*	Yes	No*
(ix) Other social benefits (school fees etc.)	No*	Yes	No*

** Not covered by (the minimum content of) an obligation of fair benefit-sharing, but potentially by other (imperfect or perfect) duties.*

in non-ideal circumstances characterized by biased or corrupt authorities. For instance, it may not be an urgent need or interest of a community to get a new soccer stadium or a *Picasso* for the research hospital lobby in return for hosting a trial. The US National Bioethics Advisory Commission (2001b, 60) demands an intrinsic connection between what people have contributed by participating in research and what is returned to them, which excludes allowing some goods completely unrelated to the provision of health care and services. The example of a soccer stadium may be extreme, but it demonstrates the point that trading off benefits can be problematic if the benefits are unrelated to the cooperative enterprise of research itself.

Yet, it should be mentioned that the vulnerability remains silent on *why* an intrinsic connection between contribution and return of benefits is needed.

They merely offer a heuristic or prudential requirement to safeguard fair benefits. The fair play model, on the other hand, fills a void in the literature, as it explains that benefits, as a matter of fairness or fair play, ought to be tied either to the intended outcome or to the intended outcome together with the research activity of a collaborative enterprise. Trading off research-related benefits in favor of other benefits lacks a normative justification.

Distributive Principles and Procedures

After having addressed the substantive content of potential fair benefits, I will now proceed to a discussion about possible principles and procedural frameworks that regulate the distribution of benefits and specify the entitlement or claim of each cooperating party. First, I should clarify that "principles of distributive justice" are (in most discussions) thought to apply to the distribution of goods resulting from economic activity (Lamont 2017a) in the national or international sphere. In view of the fair play model and the context of international health research, any valuable principle of distributive justice should identify a criterion for determining the distribution of benefits and burdens in a *pre-institutional cooperative scheme*, which is not necessarily identical with a basic structure or formal institutions. Rawls (TJ, TJR), by contrast, argues that distributive justice is primarily a concern of social schemes and their regulatory institutions (Murray 2015). Thus, the context in which different positions and principles are discussed matters. I nevertheless defend my use of the term as consistent with Rawls in so far as distributive justice applies to cooperative schemes in which goods are jointly produced and distributed.[7]

The fair play model regulates cooperative enterprises in virtue of each individual's *cooperative contribution* (burdens) and *receipt of benefits*. In this regard, fair play is compatible with desert-based principles of distributive justice. Advocates of desert-based principles argue that some agents may deserve a higher level of goods or benefits contributions even if an unequal distribution of benefits results. Most contemporary desert theorists follow the idea to guarantee to individuals the fruits of their own labor (Lamont 2017a).

These theories fall either in the category of contribution principles—which hold that people should be rewarded for their work activity according to the value of their contribution to the social product (Miller 1976, 1989; Riley 1989)—or in the category of effort principles—according to which people should be rewarded according to the effort they expend in their work activity (Lamont 2017a; Milne 1986; Sadurski 1985).

Desert-based principles, like other distributive principles (e.g., welfare-based or utilitarian principles) are *substantive* principles that appeal to a desired distributive pattern. In contrast, *procedural* principles aim to assure just procedures but do not evaluate the end-state of a distribution.[8] Many normative accounts make use of both outcome-based and procedural fairness. The economic model, for instance, proposes fair procedures (fair negotiations) to attain an end-state desert-based distribution in transactions that reflects the individual contributions made and the benefits received of each party (Emanuel and Participants 2008; Emanuel 2008; see also Chapter 3). At this point, I will discuss two further accounts that have been applied to the contexts of both health research and public health, namely, Angela Ballantyne's use of the maximin rule and adaptation of Rawls' difference principle to fair benefit-sharing and Norman Daniels and James Sabin's allocative account of "accountability for reasonableness." Regarding the latter, I will intend to transfer some of their key insights from allocative justice[9] in public health to the context of fair benefit-sharing. I will evaluate these proposals by taking into consideration the insights so far gained from the fair play model.

The Difference Principle Applied to Health Research

Ballantyne (2010a, 28) criticizes the procedural fairness account of the economic model because it does not state a clear criterion for a fair distribution of benefits. Instead, she advocates the "maximin rule" to attain a fair distribution of benefits. This requires that the benefits of cooperative activity be distributed in a manner that is to the greatest advantage to the worst-off. The maximin rule requires comparison of the minimum utility provided by each choice option and directs the chooser to maximize the minimum in decisions made under ignorance (Resnik 1987, 26).[10] Ballantyne (2010a) claims that she follows Rawls'

(TJ, TJR), who uses the maximin argument to develop principles of justice that underpin basic structures. In particular, his difference principle requires that all social institutions be arranged to maximize the expectations of the most disadvantaged in society (Rawls TJ, 75f). In other words, the difference principle permits diverging from strict equality so long as the inequalities in question would make the least advantaged in society materially better off than they would be under strict equality (Lamont 2017a). Ballantyne (2010a, 30) explicitly states that her account is in line with Rawls' difference principle, which she applies as a distributive principle to health research.

In this vein, Ballantyne (2010a) argues that benefits should be provided to the worst-off party in health research, notably host communities, as long as the transaction remains advantageous for all parties. The worst-off party is often characterized by a greater lifetime disadvantage and by significant forms of disadvantage relating to health, poverty, poor access to education, and the violation of civil and political rights (Barsdorf and Millum 2017, 108–9). However, this does not mean that sponsoring companies should be obliged to conduct research at a loss for the benefit of poor populations, as commercially outsourced research remains a voluntary enterprise. Rather, incentives for economically worthwhile commercial operations should be maintained to promote outsourcing research and the investment in LMIC health systems. Differently put, most of the benefits created through research should accrue to the worst-off while maintaining the profitability of outsourced research. Hence, Ballantyne's use of the maximin rule and her adaptation of the difference principle is especially suitable for situations of asymmetric negotiating power between the different (better- and worse-situated) parties involved in research.

However, it is crucial to note that Ballantyne seems to conflate the levels of application with regard to Rawls' difference principle too easily: while she focuses on a distributive principle in *individual* economic interactions or cooperative schemes, Rawls' principles were originally designed to regulate an *institutional (usually domestic) structure* to which individuals belong (Rawls TJ). Differently put, Ballantyne jumps from one context to the other without justifying this choice. As I previously explained, Rawls focuses on the arrangement of the basic social structure, which concerns the background circumstances regulated by socio-economic institutions (Rawls TJ, 274f).

Furthermore, and this is even more important, I argued beforehand that a basic structure model cannot be deducted in a straightforward way from the context of international health research in which agents belong *prima facie* to different basic structures.

To reply to this specific critique, Ballantyne (2010a, 31) argues that the difference principle must be considered in the global context of extreme poverty and the existence of background injustices, where the worst-off systematically lack access to even basic health care. Ballantyne concludes from this that sponsors are only permitted to benefit from the unjust and disadvantaged background circumstances if most of the surplus of the interaction accrues to the worst-off, and not to the pharmaceutical companies and populations in HICs. Hence, Ballantyne seems to derive from existing background injustices and a global health and income gap between citizens in HICs and LMICs the conclusion that research resources and spending must follow a global difference principle. This conclusion is, however, not inevitable in Rawlsian theory (Rawls TJ, TJR, LP).

As I argued in the past chapters, the fair play model is not grounded in a cosmopolitan basic structure but relies on a less demanding consideration: research constitutes a joint cooperative venture in which each party should benefit according to desert, i.e., in relation to the individual contributions to the collaborative enterprise. Existing background injustices do not automatically imply the application and imposition of a global difference principle. Rather, I argued that background injustices negatively impact the *accomplishment* of fair benefit-sharing according to the principle of fair play in a cooperative scheme.[11] But this fairness requirement does not rest on the existence of (global) unjust structures, but rather on the cooperative nature of research. However, even if Ballantye did not want to follow the fair play model, she would still need to show that a global basic structure exists to make her argument salient, which is a consideration of whether countries are institutionally and economically mutually dependent and interconnected (see Beitz 1979; Pogge 2005a). This argument, however, is *not* related to the economic and social injustices of poor countries *per se*, given that injustices can be of domestic nature, for instance, when based on an unjust resource distribution on a domestic level (see Cohen 2010, 23).

Furthermore, if globally applied, a difference principle would regulate the global basic institutional structure and not particular interactions, such as individual research trials between rich and poor agents (see Beitz 1979). I suggest Ballantyne would need to further underpin the claim that the difference principle, actually designed for a broader theory of justice, can be applied to individual health research trials (see McMillan 2010).[12] At the end of the day, principles designed for basic structures must be, if one wants to apply them to individual international health research trials, translated into principles for single (pre-institutional) cooperative schemes. Eventually, one should also note that a difference principle as a regulatory principle for the distribution of benefits cannot be easily reconciled with the basis of the fair play model. This is the case because the desert-based, that is, contribution/effort-focused, fair play model is not strictly in line with the idea to maximize the expectations of the most disadvantaged, which does not directly trace individual contributions or efforts. The difference principle exceeds the scope of fair play.

Accountability for Reasonableness

Daniels' (1996, 2000, 2008) and Sabin's (Daniels and Sabin 1997, 2002, Ch. 4) account of accountability for reasonableness is one of the most famous, applied,[13] and cited accounts for priority setting regarding the allocation of health resources under scarcity. Their account neither proposes a framework for distributive (as opposed to allocative) justice[14] in cooperative schemes, nor addresses benefit-sharing in health research. Rather, it is focused on the public health context. Even though not tailored to the context of fair benefit-sharing in health research, it seems nevertheless useful to introduce this alternative procedural meta-account, which is neither based on substantive outcomes, like Ballantyne's (2010a) account, nor adheres to fair negotiations on research markets, as defended by the economic model. The account has been widely discussed in the literature and applied to issues of fairness in research (Dupras et al. 2024; Pratt et al. 2018).

I should furthermore state that even though Daniels and Sabin's account does not particularly favor a market-fairness account—as I will further explain in the next paragraph—Emanuel et al. (2008), some of which are defenders of the economic model, are informed by Daniels' general account. More specifically, in "An Ethical Framework for Biomedical Research," Emanuel et al. (2008) say that general ethical principles regulating research and their specifications (benchmarks) can never be specific enough to eliminate controversy and deliberation. Accountability for reasonableness is then required to identify potential solutions to the problem of how to apply principles to specific cases. Daniels et al. (2000) have previously defended similar reasoning for health care reforms. Thus, I here acknowledge that Emanuel et al. and the defenders of the economic model may rely on some of the important aspects of Daniels et al.'s general theory. Despite these similarities, there remains an important difference: Daniels and Sabin (1997, 2002) reject market fairness as too narrowly conceived. This challenges the economic model, which mainly relies on Wertheimer's (1999) market account and proposes procedures related to "fair negotiations."

In what follows, I will inquire more into Daniels and Sabin's conception of *procedural fairness*, keeping in mind the question of whether it can be used as an alternative to outcome-based and procedural market accounts. As a core component of Daniels and Sabin's account, accountability for reasonableness first and foremost poses an alternative to market accountability:

> Accountability for reasonableness obviously goes beyond what is required by market accountability alone. … Accountability for reasonableness requires that we also have access to the reasons for the [an agent's or institution's] policies and decisions, and that these policies and decisions be based on the kinds of reasons fair-minded people consider relevant to the challenge of providing high quality care to all within limited resources. (Daniels and Sabin 2002, 45)

Here, Daniel and Sabin (2002) refer to market accountability as the idea that resource allocation is made according to the market choices of agents. In markets, consumers and purchasers make their decisions independently and autonomously in the light of the decisions of other agents. However, market accountability alone does not solve the legitimacy and fairness problems of distributions especially on imperfect markets or in cases of significant power differences between agents (see London and Zollman 2010). Hence, accountability for reasonableness is the idea that the reasons or rationales for important resource allocation decisions should be ones that "fair-minded" people can reasonably accept under necessary resource constraints. Fair-minded people are all those who seek to *cooperate* with one another on terms they can justify to each other and who seek for mutually acceptable rules to provide the grounds on which disputes can be adjudicated (Daniels and Sabin 1997, 2002, 43f).

Daniels and Sabin (2002, 45f) and Daniels (2008, 103f) suggest the following four conditions to render the notion of accountability for reasonableness more precise for the case of allocative justice:[15]

i. Publicity condition: Decisions and their supporting rationales must be transparent and publicly accessible;
ii. Relevance condition: Decision-makers must offer a reasonable explanation of the way in which resource allocation (distribution) decisions are made and in meeting the varied health needs of a defined population under reasonable resource constraints. Reasonable rationales appeal to evidence, reasons, and principles that are accepted as relevant by fair-minded people who aim to find mutually justifiable terms of cooperation;
iii. Revision and appeals condition: there must be mechanisms to challenge past and present resource allocation decisions;
iv. Regulative condition: there is either voluntary or public regulation to ensure (i)–(iii) are met.

The key idea of the four conditions is that fair-minded people will agree that the reasons underlying a decision are relevant to promoting health and meeting health needs fairly in the context of resource constraints, different interests, and reasonable disagreements.[16] Fair-minded people give weight to the goal of having all relevant reasons and stakeholders considered (Daniels and Sabin 2002, 63). Daniels and Sabin (2002, 48) specify that their procedural approach involves a form of reflective equilibrium, a movement between deliberation and practice, which follows to a great extent Rawls' claim that resource allocation decisions should be regarded as fair when they result from fair decision-making (Daniels 2008, 103f; see also Badano 2014; Daniels 1996; Rawls 1971). Considered judgments are reflected in past decisions and constitute relatively fixed points that serve as a basis for further deliberation and reasons. Decision-making always involves disagreement, for example, about the relative importance of the benefits and risks borne by each stakeholder. Nevertheless, there must be criteria that all stakeholders should accept as relevant and appropriate, if not sufficient, for making decisions (Daniels and Sabin 2002, 53). There should also be a commitment to giving reasons, meaning that decisions must be made in a reason- and principle-mediated way, which is publicly recognized by stakeholders. Not giving stakeholders an opportunity to understand how decisions are made deprives them of an opportunity for participating fairly in deliberation.

Daniels (1996, 2008) and Daniels and Sabin (1997, 2002) address the context of resource allocation in health care in the form of an ideal decision-making process that underlies a basic structure and an institutionalized deliberation process. Again, as I previously said, the fair play model neither presupposes a basic structure, nor relies on principles or procedures for the allocation of health resources. Fair benefit-sharing under the fair play model is first and foremost framed as a moral obligation of *distributive* fairness borne by cooperators. Nevertheless, is there a lesson to be learned from Daniels and Sabin's framework? The core intuition of accountability for reasonableness might inform the case of fair benefit-sharing in health research: without specifying outcome-based fairness, we may agree that fair play asks from stakeholders a commitment to reason-based deliberation about which benefits and burdens should enter the weighing of benefits and burdens in a cooperative enterprise.

Such a strategy is opposed to the economic and vulnerability models, the first relying on fair negotiations or market accountability, as opposed to deliberative accountability, and the latter making substantive claims about the health value of a tested intervention, as well as its availability, by ignoring deliberation and procedural fairness. Accountability for reasonableness as a meta-framework for procedural fairness, however, holds that disagreement about the precise content and magnitude of benefits and burdens as well as the translation of benefits can only be resolved when agents are fair-minded, i.e., interested in a joint goal to treat each other fairly. Fair-minded people give weight to the goal of having all relevant reasons and stakeholders considered. It is important to note that accountability for reasonableness as a meta-framework would not provide a distributive principle for fair benefit-sharing. Rather, all reasonable principles would be considered valuable options that are further subject to deliberation if stakeholders can reasonably accept them. In this sense, it can lay the procedural groundwork for fair benefit-sharing.

If we want to use Daniels and Sabin's framework, we need to adapt the four conditions to the specific context of health research and fair benefit-sharing, tailored to a decision about distributive (and as I argued) desert-based justice for all parties within the limits of a cooperative scheme. As in the original approach of accountability for reasonableness, reasonable rationales would appeal to evidence, reasons, and principles that are accepted as relevant by fair-minded people who aim to find mutually justifiable terms of cooperation. The publicity condition, i.e., transparency and publicly accessible decision-making, should offer to all stakeholders the possibility of fair and transparent participation in the decision process. The relevance condition would be a safeguard to assure the "relevance" of benefits in terms of a true health gain to a representative cross-section of the population and sub-populations, such as minorities. The relevance condition is further backed up by revisions and appeals where previous distributive decisions about benefits can be critically revised and publicly assessed.

Daniels and Sabin's approach, if adapted to benefit-sharing, seems to be in line with the general spirit of the fair play model. As the term "fair play" suggests, benefit-sharing should be subject to a cooperative process within a cooperative scheme fair-minded people can agree to. Other authors, such as Pratt and Hyder (2017), recently echoed this idea by stating that an account of distributive justice should describe a process for making decisions embedded in a deliberative process and norms, such as reasonableness, inclusion, accountability, and transparency (Pratt and Hyder 2017, 460). This has also the potential to impact the concept of community engagement (see discussion in Section "Community Engagement"; Pratt and de Vries 2018). However, to make such a vision feasible, it seems that the basic prerequisites for a fair deliberation process need to be institutionalized to safeguard fair procedures (and, in consequence, fair outcomes).

Institutionalizing Fair Benefit-Sharing?

Procedural fairness following the model of accountability for reasonableness calls for an institutional framework that guarantees publicity, relevance of arguments and reasons, and especially the possibility for revisions, appeals, and regulation. Such an institutional framework is crucial to safeguard fair procedures and outcomes. It is true that the fair play model, as conceptualized in the past three chapters, makes primarily a moral claim about fair benefit-sharing to *ground* fairness obligations, and thus abstracts from an institutional architecture necessary to attain fair benefits. Nevertheless, especially from a practical stance, it may be necessary to institutionalize the obligations of researchers and sponsors (and other agents) to make fair benefit-sharing a reality instead of only a moral aspiration. Accountability for reasonableness is a very general meta-framework for fair procedures that allows, in principle, for a variety of different institutional designs and distributive principles, on condition that fair-minded people can reasonably agree on the terms of the chosen procedures.

The fair play model, which does not rely on any prior institutional framework that appeals to a basic structure, is nevertheless in line with institutions that are tailored to *safeguarding fair benefits*. A potential institution or set of institutions designed to regulate fair benefit-sharing need not necessarily be part of background institutions regulating social schemes (see the institutional mechanisms outlined in Section "Mechanisms"). The core idea is that institutions provide mechanisms for safeguarding fair benefits and fair procedures so that fairness is sufficiently realized.

Let me outline more specifically the reasons in favor of institutionalization. In a discussion on medical innovation and the duty to contribute to generalizable knowledge, some claim that the moral burden of producing knowledge should not be placed on individual physicians but on policymakers, institutions, and public funders (Laurion and Robertson 2019). Is this also true for the case of fair benefit-sharing in international health research? I argued that any agent that (disproportionally) benefits from a research enterprise owes a fair share of the produced benefits in return to those who have restricted their liberty and contributed in a significant way to the knowledge production. So, the *moral* burden does not only fall upon policymakers, institutions, and public funders from HICs whose citizens make use of the socially valuable knowledge produced abroad but also on researchers and private sponsoring agencies that benefit from the clinical trials they conduct. Nevertheless, it is difficult, if not completely impossible, to make researchers and sponsors comply with their obligations if there is no institutional mechanism that obliges them to act on fair terms. Only institutionalized mechanisms can lead in the long run to a sustainable and significantly greater number of fair clinical trials in LMIC communities.

Moreover, a claim to a fair share in cooperative circumstances presupposes that there is an institution that specifies and assigns individual claims and obligations for all relevant stakeholders (Meckled-Garcia 2013, 83f). Failing to give people their fair share, or extracting unreasonable burdens from them, is primarily an institutional failure.[17] This is a relevant point for fair benefit-sharing in international health research: the mere fact that researchers, sponsors, host communities, and other parties join a cooperative and mutually beneficial enterprise is indeed sufficient to formulate fairness claims and obligations of the participating agents. However, (fairly designed) institutions may be needed to formulate the precise content and principles of fair benefit-sharing. Fair benefits then depend on fair institutions that enable fair deliberation among involved parties, fair reasons, and fair procedures for challenging past outcomes and improving procedures in the interest of all fair-minded stakeholders. An institutional design complying with these requirements still resembles a utopia in the context of international health research. How exactly institutions would need to be designed is a relevant question and requires an in-depth inquiry, which exceeds the scope of this book.

Mechanisms

Instead of offering a full-fledged account of possible institutionalization strategies for realizing fair procedures and outcomes, I here discuss some possible institutional mechanisms that have so far been proposed and discussed in the literature. I will analyze these proposals on the criterion of whether they can contribute to and safeguard fair procedures and the substantive content of fair benefits for host communities. This is a rough outline of some widely discussed proposals, which leaves room for new and other proposals in the future. The following mechanisms are not mutually exclusive and rival, but rather complementary to each other, and indeed may only work in conjunct implementation.

Global Research Tax

Ballantyne's (2010a) proposal of a global research tax would be, if realized, applicable to any commercial sponsor outsourcing research to developing countries. This proposal has, for instance, been further discussed as tax collected from all countries to finance vaccine research and development, as well as to ensure equitable access to vaccines in low- and middle-income countries (Albertsen 2022; Holzer and Germani et al. 2023).

In Ballantyne's original version of the proposal, researchers and sponsors would be allowed to gain benefits relative to the cost of conducting a study, and would need, at the same time, to leave a proportion of the surplus benefit to the research population. This revenue could, for instance, be used for local health-related capacity building. According to Ballantyne, the tax would be a percentage of the cost of the trial in the developing country and the appropriate tax rate would be derived from the relative costs of doing the same research in a developed country, which would provide a mechanism for distributing the surplus benefit of international research in a manner that maximizes the value for research populations in LMICs (Ballantyne 2010a, 31). This would represent a departure from other approaches, as benefit distribution in clinical trials would be defined relative to the next best alternative for researchers in HICs. Ballantyne claims that in this way the powerful party in a research interaction is required to rescue the vulnerable party or to fix the background conditions while for-profit investment in international research is not disincentivized. Research communities would maximize their interest, given that the research remains economically attractive for sponsors. A global research tax would be in addition to the existing costs of research. Thus, necessary investments in local infrastructure for the purposes of a clinical study would not be "tax deductible." A tax would be compulsory and applied equally to all commercial research sponsors conducting biomedical research in developing countries (Ballantyne 2010a, 32).

Ballantyne's (2010a) proposal has triggered a series of critiques, which concern (i) negative externalities, and (ii) practicality concerns. I will briefly outline these critiques and finally make a critical point that arises from an evaluation under the fair play model.

Regarding (i) the negative externalities of a global research tax, many authors think that a tax potentially deters research sponsors from conducting research in LMICs, as conducting research becomes more expensive and the incentive to initiate a clinical study decreases (MacDonald and Walton 2010; Resnik 2010). In the long run, they claim, a tax increases the welfare of participants in developing countries, but in the short term it may lead to a reduction in the number of trials, which potentially reduces the welfare of those who miss out. In other words, the benefits to those who gain places in the trials would increase while the number of patients and communities who make it into this pool decreases (Macklin 2010). Regarding (ii), practical concerns, Macklin (2010) as well as Schuklenk (2010) note that in order to implement a tax for research in LMICs, one would need to know with reasonable accuracy the comparative cost of conducting the trial in the developed versus the developing world and pharmaceutical companies are unlikely to release the data. Ballantyne (2010b, W6) agrees that a tax rate would only be an approximation, and a standard rate would be derived from the data available.

I will not deepen the discussion of these issues but will add an important point that arises from the perspective of fair play. Much of the discussion concerns the application of a tax under the maximin rule together with the difference principle and its practicality. Particularly, if the practicality issue mentioned (ii) is taken seriously, would curb any discussion of fair benefit-sharing, as benefits and burdens can never be calculated on a proper and ideal epistemic level but rely on real-world data. But this problem occurs in any context in which economic theory is applied in practice. Implementing a theoretical discourse is always done imperfectly and approximately.

So, the question I would like to ask is whether a global research tax is an appropriate institution or mechanism for guaranteeing fair benefit-sharing.

Or differently put, would a global research tax lead to less free- or cheap-riding on the efforts of communities? At the first glance, it seems that tax is indeed a relatively simple and well-functioning mechanism to redistribute benefits to the more vulnerable party with hypothetically less power in free negotiations, especially in circumstances where procedural mechanisms like free negotiations do not work due to market and power imbalances. Based on the empirical assumption that poor communities are very prone to being exploited, even a relatively low research tax could already significantly push the distribution toward an equilibrium of significantly more benefits for communities.

However, there is a substantive problem with the mechanism itself: a research tax consists in monetary benefits, which are *prima facie* unrelated to the benefits that emerge in the course of cooperation. Thus, there is a significant possibility that the money flow resulting from tax collection would not contribute to assuring benefits related to the cooperative enterprise, such as the provision of drugs, capacity-building, training of health personnel, and other benefits (see Section "Possible Benefits and Their Evaluation under the Fair Play Model"). Especially in non-ideal circumstances characterized by background injustices, such as economic and health inequities there is an additional risk that a tax can easily fall into the hands of few privileged people that do not have the incentive to pass benefits to the community members. Also, money is prone to being converted to "other" benefits with a very low or limited social value given the urgency of health needs. In view of these concerns, a research tax alone (without any additional content constraint on fair benefits) is not an adequate safeguard for fair benefits.

A Reformed Patent Regime

Patents are currently the most common mechanism for stimulating pharmaceutical research. They are important because companies can transform the generated socially valuable knowledge, an informational good, into profit, which incentivizes investigation. Indeed, one of the major aims in designing the current international patent agreement TRIPS was to create a reward mechanism for pharmaceutical companies to recover costs, to make profits, and, importantly, to promote research for diseases that affect developing nations (Buchanan et al. 2011; Luna and Holzer 2025; Pogge 2009). However, the TRIPS agreement exacerbated the problem of accessing medicines, as drugs are expensive under the current patent regime and unaffordable for most of the world's population (Faunce and Nasu 2008, 146; Igbokwe et al. 2022; Li and Guo 2025; Luna and Holzer 2025; WTO 2001). After the implementation of the TRIPS agreement, the generic industry for new drugs was effectively shut down in developing countries due to the strict patent protection on a global scale. Access to new innovations is effective on a twenty-year delay due to the TRIPS patent scheme. Pogge has argued that in consequence, an even higher percentage of the global poor have been excluded from drug access than in the pre-TRIPS era (Pogge 2008, 73–6, 2009, 543–6).[18]

To address this problem, Hollis (2008) and Pogge (2008, 2009) suggest a mechanism to solve the problem of access to innovative treatments and interventions (e.g., drugs, vaccines, biologicals), which would, at the same time, be useful to incentivize research on neglected diseases, such as malaria, AIDS/HIV, tuberculosis, and other tropical diseases that primarily affect LMICs. They propose a so-called "Health Impact Fund" (HIF), which offers a second patent option alongside the current patent regime (Hollis 2008; Holzer and Pogge 2020; Pogge 2008, 2009). Furthermore, the HIF has more recently been discussed by authors in the context of engaging in pharmaceutical research in the Global South (Lee et al. 2021).

Under the HIF, pharmaceutical companies that bring new drugs to market would have the option to either set monopoly prices under patents or to register new medicines with the HIF. The company could patent a drug registered with HIF in any country but would be obliged to sell it everywhere during the reward period (ten years) at a determined price, ideally at (production) cost. HIF regulations would also require companies to offer a free license of the technology needed to produce the drug after the reward period (Hollis 2008, 127). Reward payments would match the profit the firm would expect to make by setting monopoly prices. Furthermore, reward payments would be based on the global health impact of the product, which could be assessed by standardized, quantitative methods used to measure the reduction in the global burden of disease (see Gold et al. 2002).

In Hollis and Pogge's reform proposal developed nations should bear most of the costs needed to build and maintain the HIF. Hollis and Pogge consider the increased spending by affluent countries as a realistic option for prudential reasons. First, prices for pharmaceuticals would also be considerably lower in developed countries (Pogge 2005b, 192). Second, Pogge states that a "free ride" on pharmaceutical research for developing countries could show goodwill on the part of the affluent countries and enable the developing world to respond more effectively to public health problems (Pogge 2005b, 193). At the end, fairer rules understood as a reward system corresponding to health impact would generate incentives to sell the drug cheaply in order to reach more patients, and to encourage other companies to copy and sell the drug. This would substantially contribute to improving the access to medicine problem for the global poor (Pogge 2009, 549).

The HIF proposal has been heavily discussed in the past decade. Some authors have criticized the fund's practicality regarding the assessment of the health impact of a drug, the fact that public funding is provided to private companies, and reliable measurements for the global burden of disease (Buchanan et al. 2015; Faunce and Nasu 2008; Ravvin 2008). Furthermore, according to Sonderholm (2010), Hollis and Pogge's reform proposal fails to consider the need for physicians, clinics, and infrastructure for the safe and effective administration of treatments. This lack of infrastructure inhibits LMIC populations' access to medical treatments and is known as the "last mile problem."

Instead of following the discussion on the HIF's practical implications, I am more interested in evaluating whether Hollis and Pogge's proposed HIF is *in principle* a possible mechanism to facilitate fair benefit-sharing. The discussion on fair benefit-sharing does not (at least directly) address the problem of incentive-setting for the promotion of research into neglected diseases on a global level. Nevertheless, a mechanism that facilitates the creation of valuable knowledge with significant relevance for LMIC communities and, moreover, a proposal making access to new medicines significantly cheaper for these communities, is in line with the aim of shifting benefits from sponsors, researchers, and affluent nations to LMIC communities.

Health researchers and sponsors could be incentivized by translating the created knowledge into private profit, while providing the tested intervention at the cheapest possible price to host communities. Third parties, such as HICs that derive considerable benefits from drug testing and that bear an obligation to contribute fairly, would eventually finance a considerable part of the investigation. Here, the advantage is that benefits deriving from a trial conducted under an HIF regime would be directly related to the generation of socially valuable knowledge associated with the cooperative enterprise between researchers, sponsors, host communities, and other third parties.

Prior Agreements

"Prior agreements" are one of the mechanisms traditionally used to make products of successful research and other benefits following clinical trials available (Glantz et al. 1998; Macklin 2004, 171). More precisely, prior agreements, also known as "community benefit agreements," are arrangements made before a research trial begins that present a realistic plan for making effective interventions or other research benefits reasonably available to a host community after the study is completed (Page 2002). Thus, the mechanism constitutes a close follow-up of the demands of the vulnerability model (Macklin 2004). The parties that are supposed to be involved in making prior agreements typically include industry or government sponsors; host-country governments and their agencies; international agencies, such as the World Health Organization; community representatives; and relevant nongovernmental organizations.

There has been considerable skepticism about the feasibility of negotiating prior agreements, and critics have objected to making such negotiations a condition of approval for proposed research trials in LMICs (see Lie 2000). Criticism mostly concerns the delay in initiating the research, and the fact that prior agreements are not legally binding, which means they can always be breached. Macklin (2004, 173–4) responds to this critique in the following way: regarding the first obligation, populations certainly benefit more if benefits are previously spelled out despite a delay in research, compared to the situation in which all the benefits are forgone because none is made available to communities. With respect to the latter objection, it is true that responsible parties can breach prior agreements; this is true as long as such agreements are not legally binding. However, it is nonsensical to argue that prior agreements should be altogether abandoned on the premise that they can be breached. The fact that some agents do not honor them is not a good reason for eliminating such agreements and the corresponding specification of fairness obligations altogether.

I consider Macklin's (2004, 171ff) rationale for prior agreements plausible. But power imbalances among the negotiating parties, the gap between representatives of communities and communities' interests, and the potential "race to the bottom" (Chapter 3) pose real dangers to the success of prior agreements. There may be two additional safeguards to be further developed to make prior agreements a feasible mechanism for the achievement of fair benefits. On the one hand, prior agreements should, in the long run, be made using some sort of fair (institutional) procedure respecting all relevant stakeholders as equal and fair-minded parties, including parties that cannot directly participate in prior agreements, such as community members other than their representatives. This is, of course, one of the most difficult undertakings in non-ideal settings and I do not pretend to have found a solution to it. On the other hand, restrictions on the substantive content of benefits may not completely avoid but could potentially assuage the concern of community exploitation. In line with Macklin's (2004) proposal, prior agreements concern the way benefits of the knowledge gained through the cooperative enterprise of research should be distributed. This avoids trade-offs of research-related benefits for alternative benefits, a problem that arises with the economic model.

Community Engagement

Community engagement is a concept that has recently gained prominence in international health research ethics, with ethics guidelines, health authorities, and funders increasingly expecting community engagement as an integral component of the research process (CIOMS-WHO 2016, guideline 7; MacQueen et al. 2015; Pratt and de Vries 2018). Community engagement can take various forms. Unique community participation and activism occurred in the context of antiretroviral HIV treatment and its accessibility, which led to the first institutionalized community advisory boards (CABs) and the US Community Constituency Group at the National Institute of Allergy and Infectious Diseases (Fregonese 2018, 42; see Lawrence and Stewart 2016).

While earlier work seemed to focus on the establishment and functioning of community advisory boards as a mechanism to engage with communities, there is now a greater variety of practices (MacQueen 2015). For instance, in "global health research partnerships," researchers seek collaborations with their counterparts in other countries to extend their expertise, build research teams with complementary skills, and attempt to produce knowledge in a more integrative way (Murphy et al. 2015). This trend is aligned with an intentional shift toward more equal power sharing in North–South partnerships (Fregonese 2018, 42). Furthermore, according to MacQueen et al. (2015, 5), "community engagement" can describe interactions among numerous groups, of many types—from local communities to disease communities to broader social groupings like ethnic groups, or even society as a whole. This is in line with both the narrow and the broad conception of community and with my understanding that community members can be relevant stakeholders on a local and societal level in health research.

National and international bodies recognize the importance of community engagement in research. For instance, the US National Institutes of Health (NIH) support community engagement in clinical and translational research via its research networks (Fagnan et al. 2010; MacQueen et al. 2015, 1). The NIH has required community representation with presence of community advisory boards since the late 1980s and early 1990s (Fregonese 2018, 42). Similarly, international guidelines, such as CIOMS-WHO (2016), state that different sectors of a research society have a stake in a proposed research trial and should be integrated into the research process.

Community engagement is thought to be a mechanism that ensures (or increases the likelihood of) compliance with ethical principles set by international codes and research standards. Furthermore, community engagement is supposed to help ensure that a community distributes benefits fairly among its members, that activities of the local research ethics committees and field workers are supported, and that nonobvious risks are identified and managed (Fregonese 2018, 41). As the study by Kamuya et al. (2014) shows, this is not always an easy undertaking. Referring to one of the interviewees, the title of their paper ("When They See Us, It's Like They Have Seen the Benefits!") strikingly demonstrates one major difficulty: in contexts of poverty and extreme deprivation it is not easy for researchers and fieldworkers to emotionally dissociate from the demands of community members that exceed the benefits associated with the research study. To cite one of their conclusions from the study:

> Community engagement is one approach to clarifying the role and different components of research, and how it differs from routine health care. However it may be an inadequate response in a context of ... poverty. Employing FWs [fieldworkers] from the community assists with having a group who can relate to communities at a personal level, and their long term presence in the community can contribute to greater mutual understanding ... regarding what benefits are and why they are provided in research. However this is clearly an ethically and emotionally demanding position for FWs. (Kamuya et al. 2014, 13)

Building on such experiences and the history of community engagement in research and public health practice, a number of accounts have been developed to underpin the ethical goals and procedures of community engagement (see MacQueen et al. 2015). Weijer and Emanuel (2000) argue that the ethical goal of community engagement is to effectively prevent community exploitation. They recommend a variety of processes by which such protections could be realized. Emanuel and Participants (2008) then transform the concept of community engagement into what they call "collaborative partnerships," one of three principles of the economic model (Emanuel 2008). Collaborative partnerships with communities shall not only minimize community exploitation, but also increase the likelihood that research has a significant and long-lasting positive impact, and demonstrate awareness of and respect for cultural differences (Emanuel et al. 2004; MacQueen 2015). Furthermore, Dickert and Sugarman (2005) add ethical goals, such as enhanced protection, legitimacy of research, and shared responsibility, for the conduct of clinical trials. A more recent framework by King et al. (2014) emphasizes the "human infrastructure" or importance of relationships among sponsors, researchers, and communities.

However, these frameworks leave out a decisive component, that is, deliberation (Pratt and de Vries 2018). Deliberate decision-making is a core component of social justice because it is a means of realizing individuals' self-determination and development. In the research context, deliberative decision-making (the selection of projects and priorities) includes all parties who are affected by a trial and who substantially contribute to it (Pratt and de Vries 2018, 457).

Deliberation is a means of facilitating decision-making based on consensus, ensuring that all relevant groups and demographics—patients, caregivers, families, health care providers, health policymakers, and health managers—are included. This also requires a variety of levels of participation, such as decision-making shared between researchers and LMIC communities. This should include members of relevant (disadvantaged) groups and those with the power to change policy and practice to benefit them, shared decision-making rather than mere consultation, and structured deliberations and interactions to minimize the impact of power disparities between LMIC community members and researchers and sponsors (Pratt and de Vries 2018, 462).

Community engagement attempts to ensure fair benefit-sharing by providing a roadmap for procedural fairness. The central concern of procedural fairness under accountability for reasonableness is the implementation of an appropriate deliberation strategy that can be endorsed by all stakeholders. This is of special concern when it comes to safeguarding the interests of the most disadvantaged groups in terms of negotiation power in a cooperative venture. Thus, successful community engagement is a valuable strategy for safeguarding the health interests of communities, making community members active and autonomous decision-makers and cooperators in a joint research enterprise, and for identifying potential benefits and burdens for each party. Furthermore, community engagement may help transform socially valuable knowledge and other capacity-creating activities into long-term health benefits for community members. This can eventually mitigate health and economic disparities between different parties (Murphy 2015). According to Fregonese (2018, 44), successful and meaningful research cannot be conducted without appropriate community engagement. But this requires time, skills, human resources, and funding to be able to build relationships with community members.

Databases to Foster Transparency

The last of the three ethical principles of the economic model is transparency. Transparency can improve the flow of information, enabling stakeholders to get closer to a fair or ideal transaction. A population in a LMIC country is likely to be at a disadvantage regarding access to information about potential benefits and burdens relative to sponsors and researchers from HICs. Thus, to address the relative disadvantage, the economic model proposes a publicly accessible repository of all benefit agreements by populations, researchers, governments, sponsors and others, such as nongovernmental organizations. The database would include information about past clinical trials, and particularly about the negotiated benefits and burdens of each party. This shall eventually facilitate the development of a standard set of fair benefits, as information about other "deals" can be reliably traced and can serve as a benchmark (Emanuel 2008, 726).

Even though I criticized the economic model regarding its normative foundation and its framework for procedural fairness, its support of transparency is very important for an effective and successful realization of fair benefit-sharing. The mechanism of a database can render a research enterprise more transparent for all participating parties, as benchmarks for benefits and burdens can be known from historical trials. Historical data on benefits are, however, no guarantee for fairness and need to be assessed with caution. Transparency can be further fostered when persons in charge and institutions that regulate and decide on benefits are transparently managed and give public account of trials, outcomes, and benefits.

Concluding Remarks

This chapter first addressed the content specification of fair benefits and then evaluated distributive principles and procedures intended to assure that the amount of benefits accruing to each stakeholder in research is fair. Regarding the first concern, I have argued that fair benefit-sharing is concerned with the fair distribution of the benefits and burdens that are associated with research as a cooperative enterprise. The added value of the fair play model, when compared with the vulnerability model, concerns its moral justification and ability to include benefits from cooperative efforts, such as access to the created knowledge and intervention under testing, and also capacity building and infrastructural improvements related to research (Table 7.1). This leaves behind pre-fixed and "purely paternalistic" (Participants 2004, 21) requirements in favor of recognizing communities as *cooperators*. Compared with the economic model, the fair play model does not conceive of communities as stakeholders who negotiate benefits, including benefits unrelated to their cooperative efforts, which itself lacks an ethical justification. I will exemplify these points in the next chapter by reanalyzing some of the case examples introduced in Chapter 1. With respect to the latter point, a distributive principle or procedural framework that gives account of the fair play model must in some way track the relative contributions or efforts of each party as well as the benefits she receives from research. As I further argued, among current accounts of procedural fairness, Daniels and Sabin's account of accountability for reasonableness can serve as a basis to build a reasonable procedural meta-framework in which fair-minded agents deliberate on the precise content and outcomes of benefit-sharing.

Last, after discussing content, principles, and procedures, I introduced and discussed five existing institutional mechanisms for safeguarding fair benefits. I argued that while a research tax may be subject to the objection that the kinds of legitimate benefits are not sufficiently specified, a reformed patent system that aims at providing tested medicines at low prices in host countries can make a considerable contribution to the goal of fair benefit-sharing in health research. Prior agreements, community engagement with an emphasis on deliberation and community participation (as suggested by Pratt and de Vries), and databases designed to promote and sustain a transparent information flow and access to data are also valuable mechanisms for safeguarding fair benefits. These different mechanisms complement each other rather than being mutually exclusive and can and should be further complemented by future feasible proposals.

Part Four

Final Considerations

8

Discussion and Conclusion

Tying Together the Main Ideas and Major Conclusions

When I laid out the main aim of this book in Chapter 1, I outlined that I would principally discuss the fair treatment of host communities in international health research by seeking a normative account to properly address the justification and content requirement:

(i) Do researchers and sponsors bear obligations toward host communities? (Justification requirement); and
(ii) If this is the case, what is the content of these obligations? (Content requirement)

Regarding the (i) justification requirement in light of my enquiry of the past chapters, I argued that the two most prevalent transactional models in the literature, the vulnerability and economic models, fail to account for the justification requirement as neither of the two normative models offers a philosophical foundation to establish community members as stakeholders (Chapter 3). I also asserted that the core problem consists in a merely transactional conceptualization of fairness, which is most salient in the case of the economic model. In order to reply adequately to the question posed under the justification requirement—whether researchers and sponsors bear fairness obligations toward communities—the transactional models would need to convincingly show that communities are stakeholders in transactions. It certainly does not suffice to claim that communities are transactional partners: as Wertheimer (2011, 286–7) contends, the mere fact that transactions produce negative (or positive) externalities that impact community members, who are otherwise not involved in transactions, does not constitute a normative foundation permitting us to postulate that researchers and sponsors (or other agents) ought to share benefits with host communities. So, it is appropriate to say that as long as one does not explicitly show that host communities are directly exposed to unfair burdens and substantive risks or contribute to the generation of benefits in concrete transactions, there cannot be any transaction-specific obligation of fair benefit-sharing toward communities (see Andanda et al. 2013).

The fair play model—mainly developed in Chapter 4—attempts to correct for the normative void regarding the justification requirement and explains why communities are stakeholders who are morally entitled to receive fair benefits. More specifically, the fair play model relies on Robert A. Phillips' (1997) principle of stakeholder fairness, a borrowing from and adaptation of the principle of fairness or fair play associated with H.L.A. Hart (1955) and John Rawls (1964, TJ, TJR). Instead of assuming that community members are stakeholders in transactions or holding some communitarian view in which people belonging to a political community become stakeholders in virtue of their membership, I reframe health research as a collaborative scheme where stakeholders act as cooperators: Cooperators jointly benefit from and contribute to, that is, bear the burdens in a collaborative scheme. Importantly, collaborative schemes are entities in which stakeholders also nonlinearly contribute to a joint goal, which is, in the case of health research, the generation of socially valuable knowledge. So, while the transactional viewpoint abstracts from background contributions—per definition, as transactional fairness is detached from the wider context of cooperation outside the terms agreed upon between transacting partners (Emanuel and Participants 2008, 293; Wertheimer 2011, 285f)—framing health research as a cooperative scheme with the joint aim to produce socially valuable knowledge allows us to account for background contributions that are not necessarily part of specified transactions but part of a broader conceptualization of cooperation that consists of a multitude of transactions.

To be identified as stakeholders, community members need to assume the function of cooperators in the nontransactional sense. The fair play model posits that individuals have a justified claim to benefit from research once they contribute in a relevant way. This is the case when individuals significantly restrict their liberty to cooperate and have an individual causal role to contribute to a collaborative scheme while exhibiting weak unanimity with regard to the shared goal. Host community members' contributions usually consist of background contributions, such as tax payments for public goods and project-specific research funding for the maintenance of facilities and training of health workers. Host community members usually benefit when research improves public health and research systems as well as health care services. Stakeholders are identified endogenously in the fair play model: all individual agents who cooperate and contribute in the relevant sense, including background contributors, have a claim on fairly benefiting from health research. Vice versa, all individual cooperators who primarily benefit from the conduct of research, and this most notably concerns researchers and sponsors, bear an obligation to return a fair amount of benefits to the other cooperators.

Proceeding from the justification requirement, the fair play model also revisits what is currently considered to be the content of "fair benefits" and "fair procedures and mechanisms" to support benefit-sharing. This affects the (ii) content requirement, i.e., the content of the obligations to share benefits fairly, which I mainly discussed in Chapter 7. The economic model suggests fair negotiations as a sufficient procedure to attain fair benefit-sharing, while the content of benefits should be left open and be subject to the stipulations of the transacting parties (Emanuel 2008; Emanuel and Participants 2008; Participants 2004). In turn, the vulnerability model imposes strict limitations on the content of fair benefits; that is, benefits have to be associated with the medical intervention under testing as to be responsive to local health needs and priorities, and go along with the objective of assuring post-trial availability of the corresponding knowledge and interventions (CIOMS-WHO 1993, 2016; Glantz et al. 1998; London 2008; Macklin 2004a, b; Pratt and Hyder 2014; Wenner 2017; WMA 2013).

Regarding the content requirement, the fair play model seems to come close to the vulnerability model as it discards the economic model's proposal of fair negotiations together with the absence of limitations on the content of benefits. This position is most notably based on the unsuitable application of negotiations to a non-ideal context characterized by an unequal distribution of negotiation power between researchers, sponsors, and communities in low- and middle-income contexts. Furthermore, similar to the vulnerability model, the fair play model sets limits on the scope of fair benefits. However, fair play leaves room for a broader range of benefits, which also includes benefits that are related to the cooperative accomplishment of a research enterprise and potentially lead to long-lasting health improvement for community members. As a core requirement, research needs to create benefits tied to the intended outcome, that is, the generation of socially valuable knowledge or the intended outcome in conjunction with the research activity itself that is necessary to attain this outcome. This is derived from the intuition of "fair play": Research embodies a benefit-creating scheme with the main goal of producing an epistemic output of mutual value, which is moreover associated with further benefits that necessarily arise from cooperation within a joint enterprise. Such "other" benefits—in relation to the joint aim—mostly comprise capacity building or the improvement of health-related infrastructure and can be traded off with other benefits, given that the research activity is prima facie designed to produce a socially valuable outcome for all cooperating stakeholders involved.

I furthermore introduced various sub-aims related to the justification and content requirement. I would like to enumerate them briefly as well as outline my major conclusions in that respect. First, I argued that there is a supposed justification both for the vulnerability and economic model offering a normative underpinning of their respective accounts. More specifically, the fair treatment of host communities according to the fairness content and/or procedures each model proposes is morally required in order to avoid the situation where communities are exploited. There cannot be a normative foundation for community exploitation if one cherishes the idea that fairness should be framed within the transactional paradigm (Chapters 2 and 3). I then suggested that it would be more fruitful to adhere to the fair play model in order to conceptualize community exploitation. Under the fair play model, communities are exploited when the principle of stakeholder fairness is violated, or framed differently, when researchers, sponsors, and other agents free-ride on the efforts of community members to contribute to the generation of socially valuable knowledge. Expressing this thought positively, researchers and sponsors ought to comply with the obligations they acquire under the fair play model because, otherwise, they commit the moral wrong of community exploitation.

Second, one of my objectives in Chapter 4 was to rule out a strongly communitarian and Rawlsian view incorporated in the "basic structure model," which seems to be an attractive alternative to the transactional paradigm (Wenner 2018a). I provided evidence that a pre-institutional and/or pre-communitarian view would be more adequate because special relationships between sponsoring agencies, researchers, and community members mainly reside in the cooperative nature of research and not in previous relationships. Thus, even though I do not completely discard the idea that the basic structure model could be eventually further developed and adapted to international health research (Wenner 2019), I prefer to adhere to a minimalist strategy by formulating fairness obligations as moral requirements arising from cooperative (pre-institutional and pre-communitarian) interactions.

Third, I expanded the discussion of fair benefit-sharing to (affluent) agents other than researchers and sponsors. Cosmopolitan theories usually occupy this terrain by specifying cosmopolitan duties to help the global poor, borne by the affluent. There have been various attempts to translate such a general duty into more concrete moral requirements in health research, where researchers, sponsors, and other affluent agents are assigned a duty to develop local health systems and infrastructure in host communities or to initiate a global reform of research institutions (London 2005, 2008; Pogge 2002, 2005; Pogge and Laukötter 2013; Pratt and Loff 2013, 2014). However, I argued that normative models relying on cosmopolitan duties barely explain—and do not necessarily intend to explain—why the affluent bear special fairness obligations toward specific communities (see Chapter 5). I furthermore contended that the fair play model, as a valuable alternative, can be extended to include other agents, mostly citizens living in the affluent world. Fairness obligations arise when these agents willingly accept benefits and/or considerably benefit from health research trials conducted in LMICs, for instance, via functioning health systems in HICs in which medical interventions tested abroad are implemented.

Fourth, one of the major objections to the transactional view I developed in Chapter 3 is that so-called structural injustice or background injustice is not sufficiently taken into account. Structural injustice, such as poor health systems, and infrastructure and education deficits are of major concern in health research because they cause community members and research participants in developing countries to be in a worse situation when interacting with researchers and sponsors (see London and Zollman 2010). This subsequently leads more frequently to unfair outcomes in terms of (community) exploitation compared to a situation in which background injustices are absent. Even though the fair play model at first does not take into consideration structural injustice, but presents an "ideal" account for why researchers, sponsors, and other affluent agents bear fairness obligations toward communities (Chapter 4), one important aim of my work has nonetheless been to account for this non-ideal concern. Chapter 6 developed and presented an account that links structural injustice with what I called systemic exploitation (understood as either a merely transactional concept or community exploitation). I asserted that this has considerable implications concerning the formulation of responsibilities to remedy structural injustices to finally make (community) exploitation a less common practice in international health research.

The Case Examples Revisited

In view of the earlier conclusions, I would like to reassess the case studies I introduced in Chapter 1, now in view of the fair play model in comparison with the two major transactional models I extensively discussed. This first and foremost serves illustrative purposes, as I seek to show that the fair play model provides a different analysis of the case examples than the current literature suggests. Leaving aside other normative accounts, such as the basic structure and cosmopolitan models in international health research,[1] my further task will be to delineate the fair play model from the two predominant transactional models I introduced in this book.

The Havrix Trial

Remember that the major discord between adversaries and defenders of the Havrix trial is based on the following arguments. Critics, and most notably

Thai scientists, lamented in the initial planning phase of the trial that the Thai community had actually no interest or capacity nor expectation of deploying the vaccine. So, it seemed, according to them, that Thai participants were used as "testing material" for the global rich. Furthermore, sponsors would not have committed to providing the vaccine to Thailand at reduced costs. However, Emanuel and Participants (2008, 305f) claim that the Havrix trial should not be easily discarded as an "unfair" or "undue" trial. Even though the vaccine was not implemented, the trial provided the benefits of a hepatitis B vaccine for 40,000 children, the improvement of medical services and infrastructure, and most apparently, valuable capacity building for future research trials hosted in Thailand. At least, so conclude Emanuel and Participants (2008, 307), the reasonable availability requirement alone should be discarded when assessing health research trials.

So, who is right? The vulnerability model has a clear answer: As testing the Havrix vaccine neither addressed an urgent local health priority of the Thai population nor was there a commitment to make the vaccine reasonably available after the trial, host communities were not treated fairly. Differently put, the trial was not in accordance with (at least) the reasonable availability requirement and (probably) the requirement to address local health needs and priorities (CIOMS-WHO 1993, 2016; Macklin 2004a,b, 2011; WMA 2013). Furthermore, as adversaries of the trial criticized, there was insufficient technology transfer, and, in particular, no training of Thai researchers regarding laboratory skills (Hawkins and Emanuel 2008, chap. 2; see Chapter 1).

Regarding the economic model, it is clear that the analysis of the Havrix trial does not easily draw us to this unambiguous answer. We would need more information about the negotiation conditions and the relative value of benefits and burdens the Thai community obtained or had to bear in order to assess whether fair benefit-sharing was achieved. Emanuel and Participants (2008, 303f) make an attempt to weigh the various benefits at stake. Even though the reasonable availability requirement was not fulfilled, there were considerable benefits, such as the modernization of infrastructure and a public health benefit through the hepatitis B vaccine. The trial, furthermore, fulfilled the background requirements of (general) social value and fair subject selection while showing a favorable risk-benefit ratio, as hepatitis A was still a (even though not pressing) health problem in Northern Thailand. There were extensive community consultations in Kamphaeng Phet province prior to conducting the trial (Emanuel and Participants 2008, 305). Eventually, defenders of the economic model claim that one would need to use a multifaceted analysis under the three principles—fair benefits, collaborative partnership, and transparency—to offer a more well-rounded analysis of the trial (Emanuel and Participants 2008, 307).

The fair play model, suggesting a different stance on fair benefit-sharing, coincides with the major conclusion of the vulnerability model. It seems that the major aim to test a vaccine in a joint research enterprise, i.e., the goal of producing valuable knowledge about whether the Havrix vaccine worked in terms of safety and efficacy, solely benefited citizens and the military of the United States and other developed countries. In this sense, it is true that an ultimate moral justification to conduct this trial in Thailand was not given. A valuable justification would have made all cooperators in the process of knowledge production subject to a fair participation in the intended epistemic output.

However, the fair play model draws a more complete picture than the vulnerability model: Benefits arising from cooperation in the Havrix trial were significant. This concerns not only the improvement of infrastructure, public health, and health services, but most importantly the intended capacity building to strengthen the local health and research system. Whether this objective was achieved remains ambiguous (Hawkins and Emanuel 2008, 58). However, if it is true that the knowledge creation in the sense of capacity building could have been, even if not the main, a considerable secondary goal, the charge of community exploitation—even though not off the table—can be considerably mitigated. So, following the fair play model, we may finally contend that researchers, sponsors, and beneficiaries from Western countries committed the wrong of "cheap riding" on the Thai community. This is a position in between the economic model that does not seem to press charges of community exploitation, and the vulnerability model that puts forward a strict notion of community exploitation based on the reasonable availability requirement without further considering valuable benefits that certainly have arisen from cooperation in the Havrix trial. Hence, the fair play model sets up the conceptual groundwork to avoid a dichotomous view between "condemnable exploitation" and "true fairness."

African HIV Maternal Transmission Trials

Calling to mind Glantz et al.'s (1998) opposition to the HIV transmission studies in the 1990s, in which a lower AZT regime than the standard 076 regimen was tested in several African countries, the main concern was that the research question was of little or no value to the host communities involved (see Chapters 1 and 2; Hawkins and Emanuel 2008, 1–2). The information derived from the studies, in particular that an AZT regime costing $50 is as effective as the expensive 076 regimen of $800–1000 per treated woman, solely benefited the developed world but not countries whose annual health expenditure per person was lower than $50. Under the vulnerability model, the charge of exploitation seems clear: Even though the treatment under testing was indeed thought to address an urgent local health need, the research question failed to be responsive to the particular low-income context. If Glantz et al. (1998) were right, the research question would never have led to a reasonable provision of the tested intervention owing to the high costs the intervention would have implied for the participating countries.

It seems the economic model would have taken into consideration the benefits that were created during the trials for the research participants; that is, at least half of the children (in placebo-controlled trials) had the potential chance to be saved from an HIV infection. Casting aside the debate regarding a double standard (Chapters 1, 2, and 6), this may not have been sufficient to prevent community exploitation, even under the economic model, as communities did not derive sufficient benefits (Hawkins and Emanuel 2008, 3). The fair play model eventually also accounts for the HIV transmission studies as exploitative, given that research as a cooperative scheme would not have produced knowledge in any relevant sense for the communities. Considering that the cooperative joint purpose of engaging in research coincides with the production of a valuable epistemic output for all cooperators, presented as the core normative requirement of the fair play model, the HIV transmission studies did not comply with stakeholder fairness. Thus, it finally seems that different models—here, the two transactional models and the fair play model—would come to the same conclusion regarding the ethics of fair benefit-sharing in the HIV transmission studies. Yet, they reach the same conclusion following different conceptual pathways, or, to express it with Derek Parfit's (2011) metaphor, the models converge rather than disagree by climbing the same mountain on different sides.

Dengue Vaccine Development and HIV Pre-exposure Prophylaxis

Regarding the current case example outlined in Chapter 1, the testing of dengue leads to similar results as seen in the first case example, the Havrix trial. The ethical concern is that the dengue vaccine, and the valuable knowledge it generates, will be accessible primarily in affluent countries and not in the countries where the drugs were tested. Under the vulnerability model, this violates the requirement of reasonable availability in the countries hosting the trials, although local health needs and priorities are adequately addressed, as dengue remains a pressing health issue in the Global South (CIOMS-WHO 1993, 2016; WMA 2013).

Similarly, the fair play principle appears to be violated: affluent sponsors and affluent populations disproportionately benefit from dengue vaccine research conducted abroad, as they gain access to the vaccines in their own countries. Even if research is accompanied by capacity building, knowledge transfer to local researchers and their facilities, and infrastructure improvements, the accusation of "cheap riding" seems to remain: a huge part of the potential benefits would consist in the access to the tested vaccines for the wider population, not just the research participants. But in the case outlined, it seems that collaboration for knowledge production only benefits the pharmaceutical industry and populations abroad and not the host communities.

This problem is compounded by two factors. First, poor countries in Latin America and Asia bear a significant health burden from tropical diseases such as dengue and would benefit greatly from the availability of preventive measures

(Tully and Griffiths 2021). However, at least for Latin America, Homedes and Ugalde (2016) have shown that countries in the region and their communities have, in the past, not benefited enough from drug testing in general. This shortcoming is evident in the lack of affordability of medicines due to high pricing regimes, which exclude the poorest individuals of the host countries from access to these medicines. In addition, poor drug registration processes further exacerbate the problem in Latin American countries (Homedes and Ugalde 2016, 228f; Chapter 1).

Secondly, this example highlights another aspect of the global justice debate that intersects with health research: the equitable global distribution of the burdens of climate change and the obligations of wealthy countries to help the Global South adapt to climate-related challenges. Because dengue is a climate change-related disease, addressing it is a health priority in the most affected regions. This urgency is compounded by the increasing threat of climate change, which is steadily expanding the geographic range of the disease and exacerbating its long-term burden in vulnerable regions (George et al. 2024; Global Forum on Bioethics in Research 2024).

The economic model applied in this case may appear more tolerant of drug trials that do not meet the reasonable availability requirement. However, it would still likely object to research conducted in the Global South where host communities do not benefit in a sustainable and long-term way. At the same time, the dengue case calls for a thorough assessment of local conditions within research communities. While there are probably notable benefits such as knowledge transfer through researcher training and infrastructure improvements and substantial benefits to research participants—given that dengue is a critical health issue in these regions—further evidence is needed to determine the extent of additional benefits.

Regarding the case of providing Lenacapavir as an HIV pre-exposure prophylaxis drug in LMICs. Recall that the Access to Medicines Foundation (2025) mourned that the laboratory *Gilead Sciences* did not guarantee the access of its tested drugs to those LMICs that have the greatest health needs because they were excluded from the license. This last case may be of particular interest to the reader because, in light of the book's discussion, it differs from the others: it advances a cosmopolitan claim about global justice, namely that a highly beneficial drug for a widespread disease should be made available to the poorest populations. Now, we may dissect this and look at what type of obligation is touched.

In a first instance, neither of the vulnerability, economic model, and the fair play model requires in terms of *special obligations* that benefits ought to be shared with communities where the research is not conducted. Differently put, special obligations of fair benefit-sharing can only be claimed where special and perfect obligations can be justified (compare O'Neill 1996). In the Lenacapavir case, testing sides were in Uganda and South Africa, and Latin America, including sites in Argentina, Brazil, Mexico, and Peru as well as the United States. Those countries could, under all normative models outlined, make claims about the provision of benefits. However, it seems the moral issue at state proclaimed by the Access to medicines Foundation is different. The claim is that the laboratory *Gilead Sciences* should be responsible to remedying a global justice issue. Now, of course, this falls under what we discussed in Chapter 5: a cosmopolitan duty of justice and the many interpretational options of how such a duty can be grounded or applied. For instance, considering an imperfect duty of beneficence, we could say that *Gilead Sciences* is in a very good position, for instance, to help global poor communities in LMICs with the greatest health needs through a nonexclusive voluntary licensing (see Millum 2011). But this cannot be conceived as a special obligation. Also, there might be more actors involved in resolving this issue, and it might be morally supererogatory for a single company to be charged the burden of global justice. To name some possible cosmopolitan routes to go: there are actors responsible for reforming the global systems of patents and licenses in international cooperation, also making clear the rules that apply for drugs with a huge potential for reducing the disease burden. In a way, Pogge and Holis' health impact fund argue that this incentive system for global research must be changed completely. Such approaches, as we saw in the last chapter, are accompanied by the idea of redistribution through a research tax—using the money to make the drug later on available in poorer countries. Last, there might be very wealthy actors from HICs who could fund the access to drugs for the poorest (e.g., through philanthropy). In short, in this cosmopolitan problematic, it seems duties of justice can be expanded and rediscussed considerably beyond special obligations benefit-sharing.

Regarding the case of providing *Lenacapavir* as an HIV pre-exposure prophylaxis drug in LMICs, recall that the Access to Medicines Foundation (2025) noted that *Gilead Sciences* did not guarantee access to its tested drugs for those LMICs with the greatest health needs because they were excluded from a voluntary license. This case may be particularly interesting to the reader because, in light of the book's discussion, it differs from the other cases: there is a cosmopolitan claim about global justice—namely, that a highly beneficial drug addressing a global disease burden should be made available to the poorest populations.

We can now dissect this case and examine what type of obligation is involved. At first glance, neither the vulnerability, economic model, nor fair play model requires, in terms of special obligations, that benefits be shared with communities where the research was not conducted. In other words, special obligations of fair benefit sharing can only be claimed where special and perfect obligations can be justified (see O'Neill 1996). In the *Lenacapavir* case, the trials were conducted in Uganda and South Africa, as well as in Latin America, including sites in Argentina, Brazil, Mexico, and Peru, as well as the United States. Those countries could, under all normative models outlined, legitimately make claims about the provision of benefits.

However, the moral issue highlighted by the Access to Medicines Foundation (2025) appears to be different. The claim is that *Gilead Sciences* should be responsible for addressing a global justice issue. This falls under the discussion in Chapter 5 regarding a cosmopolitan duty of justice and the various interpretational options for grounding or applying such a duty. For instance, considering an imperfect duty of beneficence, we could think that *Gilead Sciences* is in a strong position to assist poor communities in LMICs with the greatest health needs through nonexclusive voluntary licensing (see, e.g., Millum 2011). Yet this cannot be conceived as a special obligation.

Moreover, multiple actors could be in a good position to address the disease burden of HIV, and it may be insufficient and unjustified to place the entire moral burden of global health justice on a single company. Possible cosmopolitan approaches could imply:

- Reforming global patent and licensing systems through international cooperation, establishing clear rules for drugs with significant potential to reduce disease burdens.
- As argued by Hollis (2007), the international community could pledge for a reformed patent system to restructure incentives for global research. Such approaches, as discussed in the previous chapter, could also be accompanied by redistribution mechanisms, such as a research tax, to ensure later availability of drugs in poorer countries.
- Wealthy actors in high-income countries could also fund access to drugs for the poorest populations (e.g., through philanthropy).

In short, in this cosmopolitan context, duties of justice can be expanded and reconsidered well beyond the framework of special obligations and benefit-sharing.

Concluding Remarks Regarding the Case Examples

The first selected case examples, the historical cases and the dengue vaccine development, served as an illustration to address the key ethical challenges in international health research with respect to the fair treatment of host communities conceived as a special obligation.[2] I aimed to guide the reader step by step through the history of research ethics in this regard, commencing with the double-standard discussions to finally reach the main subject matter, i.e., fair benefit-sharing with host communities. As much of the debate commenced with the earlier-mentioned cases and, most conspicuously, with the HIV transmission studies triggering a whole series of papers and discussions, I also considered it to be crucial to address "old" concerns and "old cases" in light of a re-interpretation and re-consideration of the underlying theoretical arguments. And as we have seen in the recent case of the dengue vaccine trials, these old concerns continue into the immediate future and still raise the same ethical questions. This, of course, is one moral concern related to global health research. As the case of HIV pre-exposure prophylaxis shows, another concern—beyond the scope of this book—is determining which agents bear responsibility for addressing global health justice and the still devastating global disease burden.

At that point, I would not only like to emphasize that the fair play model alters the analysis of (some of) the case examples, as demonstrated previously, but also that fair play offers a valuable inclusion criterion for community members as stakeholders in health research as a collective enterprise. With a detailed argument in Chapter 4, I consider community members as stakeholders that hold a valid claim to receive fair benefits as long as they act as collaborators in the relevant fashion, that is, as long as they at least contribute in the background to the production of socially valuable knowledge. As I alluded to in Chapter 1, the outlined case examples and many debates conceive of communities as host countries. I later on argued that citizens of host countries can be attributed a cooperative role in health research as long as they bear the burdens when making background contributions, such as tax payments to provide and maintain research facilities and education of health workers. It is certainly the case that local communities, such as, for instance, the local community in Kamphaeng Phet, in which the Havrix trial was conducted, are more closely involved in and affected by a research enterprise than the wider political community of a country. This is true when health personnel are withdrawn from the local health system, like hospitals, and employed in the research enterprise or when economic and social resources are directly drawn from local sites. However, this does not mean that members of the wider political community of a host country cannot be established as stakeholders in a wider collaborative scheme via background contributions. Members and contributors of such a wider scheme might have a claim on fewer benefits, but yet a certain amount of benefits may be owed to them.

General Objections and Replies to the Framework

The fair play model is intended to provide a workable framework to make sense of the concepts and arguments that have been brought forward in international health research ethics, dating back to the late 1980s and early 1990s, and continuing to this day. I have, however, so far ignored several critical lines of contentions that can be brought forward and indeed were brought forward against certain aspects of the concept of fair benefit-sharing itself.

Before moving to the concluding remarks, I would like to outline and discuss two general and important critiques concerning the concept of fair benefit-sharing drawn from the current research ethics literature. These critiques relate to, first, a non-ideal objection; that is, there is a moral cost of applying ethical principles to real-world contexts. As briefly mentioned in Chapter 6, Wertheimer (1999, 289–93, 2011, 2012) repeatedly emphasized that our moral considerations have to be contextualized in the real world in order to prevent us from bringing about worse ethical outcomes than in a status quo *ex ante*. I will discuss this concern under the label of the "non-worseness claim." Second, there is a general concern toward any kind of benefit-sharing related to the danger that communities may be "unduly" incentivized to participate in and support a research project because of the mere receipt of benefits. This concern is commonly known as "undue inducement."

First Objection: Fair Benefits and the "Non-Worseness Claim"

The non-worseness claim states that an interaction between A and B cannot be morally worse than no interaction at all if A and B are both better off, compared to a baseline of no interaction (Malmqvist 2017, 478). Wertheimer (2011, 256ff) has used this argument to say that third parties, such as regulatory agencies, governments, or research ethics committees, should not prevent Pareto-superior transactions, including mutually beneficial exploitation, on the grounds that they are unfair.[3] This is a non-ideal objection taking into consideration that researchers and sponsors in the real world are noncompliers with ethical standards and principles, such as certain fairness standards set by normative models. This is of relevance for fair benefit-sharing with host communities. It can be generally assumed that "fair trials" according to a valuable fairness criterion, such as stakeholder fairness in the fair play model or transactional fairness in the economic model, are more expensive compared to "unfair trials" (Macklin 2004a). The reason behind this is simply that a greater share of the benefits in a research enterprise accruing to host societies goes along with augmented costs for researchers, sponsors, and other agents who are placed under an obligation to provide these benefits.

Note that Wertheimer's argument points to the situation in which banning exploitative research implies that researchers and sponsors have reasons to forgo mutually beneficial trials and relocate them to other (high-income) countries. One possibility to avoid the non-worseness claim within the economic model rests on the strategic argument. Wertheimer (2008, 81) says in what he calls the "strategic argument" that regulators may have favorable reasons to prohibit exploitative transactions if this (still) incentivizes parties to engage in fair transactions. Thus, if we have favorable reasons to assume that the amount of mutually beneficial transactions does not (significantly) decrease under regulations that prohibit exploitation, we ought to pursue this strategy.

The non-worseness claim, if true, is, however, a very relevant constraint concerning fair play in joint enterprises that are set up together with communities. Wertheimer's point is relevant because it similarly impacts the practice of allowing for research trials that do not comply with fair benefit-sharing in non-ideal circumstances. However, some scholars argue that the non-worseness claim can be mitigated (even if this implies neglect, i.e., fewer research trials that potentially benefit the global poor). As I outlined in Chapter 6, Malmqvist (2017, 484) makes this attempt and contends that researchers and sponsors take advantage of injustice when they exploit (which is independently wrong from exploitation). They furthermore act as accomplices insofar as they foreseeably contribute to the maintenance of structural injustices of which they take advantage when they exploit and send the message that those primarily responsible for background injustices are not morally required to remediate them.

Expanding on that, I argued that we might have strong reasons to ban what I called systemic exploitation—exploitation (probabilistically) caused by background injustice—if we want to follow the premise that exploitative practices themselves enable, foster, and maintain unjust background conditions and that this, in turn, makes systemic exploitation itself more likely. Put another way, if banning exploitation contributes to less background injustice in the long run, which reduces the exploitation rate, we will have reasons to believe that the non-worseness claim can be considerably mitigated: banning exploitation leads to fewer exploitative acts in the long run. Yet, we should not forget that this comes with costs for research subjects and communities in the short run as potential benefits are forgone.

I contended that community exploitation is systemic. Following this previous argument, the prohibition of clinical trials not complying with stakeholder fairness may contribute to the remediation of background injustices in the long run (Chapter 6). In particular, a prohibition would place (economic and ethical) pressure on responsible agents to remedy background injustices. This, in turn, would form a new basis to conduct fairer clinical trials in the developing world. I asserted in Chapter 6 that this line of argument needs to be empirically validated. Structural background conditions are complex clusters of socioeconomic factors. The remediation of background conditions might need to be performed in a very significant way, including the introduction of health care coverage for a considerable cross-section of a potential research population, to let community members fairly benefit from research.

Yet, apart from these considerations, does Wertheimer's non-ideal objection—if based on the correct premise (that researchers and sponsors forgo mutually beneficial trials if they are too expensive)—pose an objection to the fair play model itself? Wertheimer's non-worseness claim is a valid concern and of major relevance in non-ideal circumstances with noncompliers, and gives guidance for regulatory agencies. However, the core of the fair play model abstracts (i) from non-ideal circumstances and (ii) even more importantly does not include guidance for the regulatory dimension of health research. Regarding (i), (non-)ideal theory, the fair play model pursues and develops an ideal fairness norm.[4] Speaking with Rawls (TJR, JF), non-ideal theorists require a benchmark of fairness, which is determined within ideal theory, in order to establish whether an action, in this case, the carrying out of clinical research, exploits host communities (Chapter 4). As Wertheimer (2011, 191f, 256f) admits, researchers and sponsors (and other agents) are not morally allowed to exploit, even in non-ideal circumstances. Then, the non-worseness claim is a secondary argument that analyzes what third parties ought to do given that researchers and sponsors act as noncompliers.

In a nutshell, the fair play model first and foremost determines the terrain of moral action (Chapters 4 and 5) prior to looking at moral guidance for third parties under non-ideal circumstances. In Chapter 6, I eventually take non-ideal circumstances into account on a structural level in relation to background injustices. This means, however, that I do not give a final answer regarding the non-worseness claim as the relation between exploitation and structural injustice in the long run needs to be further (empirically) specified. As argued above, whether the earlier argument—that the prohibition of exploitation leads to less structural injustice and exploitation in the long run—holds in real-world circumstances must be further discussed.

Regarding (ii), I developed and outlined the pillars of fair play and ignored so far the regulatory dimension of fair benefit-sharing. However, as Laurion and Robertson (2019) convincingly argue, policymakers, institutions, and public funders need to make certain that moral requirements are institutionalized. It is impossible to make researchers and sponsors comply with fairness obligations in the real world if there is no institutional mechanism that constrains them to act on fair terms. Institutionalization further downstream would eventually need to provide a specific answer to whether (hugely) exploitative research should be banned or not. Here, Chapter 7 presented some concepts and ideas of how to proceed in terms of regulation, institutionalization, and mechanisms with the goal of turning researchers, sponsors, and affluent agents into compliers. Even though I did not address the non-worseness claim, one of the major conclusions was that procedures, institutionalization, and mechanisms adhering to the core concern of the fair play model must be based on a reasonable procedural meta-framework in which fair-minded agents deliberate on the precise content, principles, and outcomes of benefit-sharing. So, it is safe to say that outcomes must be in line with what fair-mindedness would require. Fair-mindedness presupposes that benefits from (even exploitative) research in the short run be weighed with benefits in the long run.

Second Objection: Undue Inducements

Many define an undue inducement in research as an offer "so attractive that it seduces people to accept it against their better judgment" (Emanuel 2004; Grant and Sugarman 2004). Payments to research subjects are typically thought to be acceptable if they are intended to reimburse subjects for financial losses incurred through research participation. However, there are payments, argue various commentators, that are offered as independent incentives to participate in research rather than reimbursement for costs incurred. Such payments should be considered "undue" when they negatively influence the judgment of potential research subjects and undermine the voluntariness of the subjects' consent (Ballantyne 2008; Macklin 1981; Wilkinson and Moore 1997). Here, the general fear, according to Ballantyne (2008, 184), is that "potential participants would be 'blinded' by the offer of money and might, therefore, underestimate the risks of research, overestimate the benefit of the cash payment or adequately weigh the risks but decide to act against their best interests in order to access the payment." To prevent this, the CIOMS-WHO guidelines (2016, paragraph 13) state that "[c]ompensation must not be so large as to induce potential participants to consent to participate in the research against their better judgment."

Undue inducements in health research are generally discussed and analyzed as monetary benefits for individual research subjects, and not necessarily as a standard problem of outsourced research in LMIC (Ballantyne 2008, 185). However, the discussion has been expanded to nonmonetary therapeutic inducements (Lee 2019) and low- and middle-income contexts, in which therapeutic benefits pose the primary incentive to participants and not financial reward (Ballantyne 2008).

According to various commentators (Macklin 1981; Wilkinson and Moore 1997), there is an inherent tension between exploitation and undue inducement. The paternalistic claim against inducements is that they will encourage research subjects to volunteer against their best interest. While undue benefits, payments, or therapeutic incentives do not represent an undue inducement per se, it is more likely that they result in undue inducements in contexts where other standard measures designed to protect, such as informed consent and just patient selection, are less stringently enforced (Dresser 2001; Emanuel 2004). This is especially relevant for international health research where patients live in non-ideal circumstances characterized by significant background injustices. This leads, especially in low-income contexts, to a paradox: The most vulnerable are entitled to benefits because they would be otherwise exploited, but those benefits may, at the same time, unduly induce them to participate. This, in turn, would morally entitle researchers and sponsors to limit the benefits they provide to trial participants.

Emanuel (2004), Ballentyne (2008), Savulescu (2001), and also Lee (2019) feel that this is no valid argument. For instance, Emanuel (2004, 104) and Savulescu (2001, 3) believe that "undue inducement" is often employed as a euphemism or instrument for paternalism, derogation, or exploitation. Kamuya et al. (2014, 13) empirically back up this claim by showing that researchers in their Kenyan field study felt that undue inducement arguments were sometimes used to reduce or deny participants' benefits. Another critique brought forward is that there is a substantive problem related to the diverse cultural and economic backgrounds potential research participants have: whether some people volunteer against their better judgment depends on their personal situation. An unemployed person or a student may view compensation differently from an employed person, which must be taken into account by research ethics committees (CIOMS-WHO 2016, 54).

For now, let us assume for the purpose of further discussion that the concept of undue inducement indeed poses a certain ethical danger in health research. My question is now whether this concern is of importance when it comes to fair benefit-sharing with community members other than research subjects. Much has been written on research subjects being unduly induced—and just very little about the potential danger of unduly inducing communities. However, even though the term "undue inducement" is a term tailored to a moral wrong imposed upon research subjects, the problem can easily be transferred to host communities, just as follows.

As the National Bioethics Advisory Commission (2001b, 60) demands, there must be an intrinsic connection between what people (or communities) have contributed by participating in research and what is returned to them, which excludes allowing a number of goods completely unrelated to the provision of health care services (see Chapter 7). This statement hints at the potential danger that communities may be unduly induced by the reception of goods "unrelated to health research," such as soccer stadiums or new schools, "blinding" them when it comes to hosting research. Yet, considering the arguments in the discussion on research subjects, it moreover seems that undue inducement not only involves "soccer stadiums" but also benefits related to treatment and cure of health conditions prevalent in a host community (Emanuel and Participants 2008; Chapter 3). In view of these concerns, the ethical models for fair benefit-sharing so far introduced owe an answer to the question of whether fair benefit-sharing implies the danger of undue inducements.

Regarding the normative models so far presented, it seems that the economic model has the least to offer as a safeguard against undue inducement. This can be explained, in part, by the intentionally "non-paternalistic" normative view (Emanuel and Participants 2008; Participants 2004). When communities "freely" negotiate and accept benefits "in their best interest," there is no "paternalistic hindrance" to obtain any (also undue) desired benefit. However, I shall note, to be fair, that Emanuel (2004), as one of the major defenders of the economic model, thinks that concerns about undue inducement[5] should be "ended" once we guarantee for trials that comply with core ethical requirements of research, not being overly risky or unjust (Emanuel 2004, 104; Emanuel et al. 2000; Emanuel et al. 2004). I shall also note that the principles of collaborative partnerships and transparency—two of the three principles of the economic model—are considered to assure fair and transparent negotiations and can therefore be considered safeguards against undue inducement.

Interestingly, Emanuel and Participants (2008, 297–8) nevertheless warn that the requirements of the vulnerability model, and especially the reasonable availability requirement, can easily lead to "undue inducement," meaning that deprived populations enroll in excessively risky research to obtain promised health benefits (see Chapter 3, Table 3). This is related to the worry that the reasonable availability of drugs is a pressing need in deprived populations, where access to public health measures, routine vaccines, medications for common ailments, and even trained health care personnel is missing. It is prima facie certainly true that deprived populations are more likely to accept excessively risky or undue research in the prospect of significant health improvements. However, this applies to any other (negotiated) benefit as well, such as schools and infrastructure projects, and, in particular, monetary benefits (Ledford 2014).

So, it seems at a general level that undue inducement is a danger in contexts of weak research regulation, as unethical research conduct is more likely, and furthermore, in circumstances of substantive background injustices, as communities are more dependent on international researchers and sponsors who potentially ameliorate the state of deprivation. Community engagement certainly constitutes one valuable approach to clarify the role of research, especially in a context of poverty. For instance, "fair rules" and generally the notion of what should be conceived as a "valid benefit" can be explained as to prevent undue inducement. Nevertheless, one shall not forget that in reality, as empirical evidence shows, adequate ethical behavior needs to be contextualized. For instance, some researchers in Kamuya's et al. (2014, 13) study argued that, in certain situations, concerns of undue inducement (here of research subjects) were perceived to be too narrow when faced with poverty and famine. Thus, it seems that strict and pre-fixed rules regarding benefit-sharing can also be counterproductive.

Eventually, there remains the question of whether the fair play model and my general discussion are able to bring forward a convincing safeguard against undue inducements. Two points on this. First, the fair play model makes benefits subject to cooperation for a joint aim. It seems the reasonable availability requirement shows the tendency to turn communities into passive bystanders that "allow" researchers and sponsors to conduct research and expect health benefits in return. In some way, the economic model seems more dynamic and involves communities and their representatives as negotiators. However, it still seems that benefits are unrelated to a joint cooperative enterprise and serve a "compensatory" hidden agenda, where burdens communities bear are compensated by "showering" communities with benefits. Undue inducements are a concern, as compensatory benefits offered by researchers and sponsors may easily overshadow how affluent agents derive valuable benefits from a research question while communities are left empty-handed in this respect.

The fair play model, in turn, makes clear that community members are not passive bystanders or negotiators but fully acknowledged contributors in a collaborative scheme. A collaborative scheme implying obligations and claims on benefits further presupposes just cooperation and a just end (Chapter 4). In this regard, fair benefit-sharing is the moral imperative to jointly produce and share the benefits from a just enterprise. This moral imperative, per se, does not entail the risk of undue inducement: Communities should be accrued a fair share of their cooperative efforts in a fair cooperative scheme. Here, they should neither be passive bystanders nor subject to negotiation procedures that are potentially related to undue benefits.

I am aware of the fact that this is a purely theoretical answer, not reflecting poor research regulations, poverty, and deprivation in LMIC research. So, second, as I repeatedly said, I intended to account for this non-ideal perspective in this work. I provided evidence that one would need to complement an account of benefit-sharing (and community exploitation) by a framework addressing pressing background injustices. More specifically, I claimed that all agents that can be held responsible should remedy background injustices to make fair benefit-sharing a more likely outcome of international health research. This, of course, would also reduce the danger of undue inducements, as communities in less precarious situations would depend less on the goodwill and help of affluent agents. Furthermore, and apart from this structural perspective—an issue that can only be addressed in the long run—Chapter 7 outlined and discussed possible mechanisms that are thought to safeguard fair benefits and just collaboration while minimizing the risk of undue inducements in current non-ideal circumstances. As previously mentioned, community engagement is one central mechanism. Furthermore, prior arrangements and databases to foster transparency may similarly be useful in this respect.

Closing Remarks

My book departed from a historical reconstruction of arguments brought forward in the debate on the fair treatment of host communities. Constructing my research question, I argued that a new normative model for fair benefit-sharing needed to be developed as an alternative to the existing ones. I first and foremost dedicated a great part of my elaborations to the normative groundwork by criticizing prevalent and popular normative models in the literature and by suggesting an alternative, the fair play model. I finally sketched and critically discussed possible distributive principles, procedures, and mechanisms to safeguard fair benefits that have so far been presented in the academic literature.

I hope to have made especially theoretical progress and offered a valuable contribution regarding the normative foundation of fair benefit-sharing. Admittedly, the fair play model could not possibly solve all real-world problems related to this concept. Even though my work addressed pressing non-ideal problems—that of background injustices prevalent in LMICs and power imbalances in negotiations between researchers with their sponsors and host community representatives—more theoretical and empirical work needs to be carried out to advance the institutionalization process and mechanisms to safeguard fair benefits for host communities. Here, the fair play model may serve as a workable normative basis to further shape these advancements. Finally, my account may also serve to complement future lines of research concerning a more general debate on global justice (other than justice in health research) and particularly the interaction between transnationally operating actors and LMICs.

Notes

Chapter 1

1 The US Food and Drug Administration (FDA) is a federal agency of the United States Department of Health and Human Services responsible for the control and supervision of food safety, tobacco products, pharmaceutical drugs, medical devices, and other medical interventions impacting public health (https://www.fda.gov/home).

2 The ICH project brought experts, in particular from the United States, Western Europe, and Japan, to create the Good Clinical Practice (GCP) guidelines as international ethical and scientific quality control standard for assuring the protection of subjects and, most notably, for guaranteeing the credibility of data. Most importantly for the clinical trials industry, ICH-GCP standards made clinical data obtained at international research sites transferable and reliable. New drugs could be more easily registered in different countries and markets could be opened globally (Petryna 2009, 35).

3 Members of the World Trade Organization (WTO) negotiated the Agreement on Trade-Related Aspects of Intellectual Property Rights (TRIPS) in the 1986–94 Uruguay Round of multi lateral trade negotiations. In a nutshell, the agreement demands that standard types of intellectual property (trademarks, designs, patents, trade secrets, etc.) be recognized and effectively protected through national law, independently of whether the intellectual property right holder is a citizen of the respective country or not (Andanda 2013, 40).

4 As I will show in Section "Examples of Current Clinical Research and Sponsorship in LMICs," tropical diseases like Dengue may become more frequent in the Global North due to climate change. As I will argue further, this can, of course, increase the efforts by high-income countries to invest in drugs for diseases that have so far been most prevalent in the Global South.

5 For a detailed introduction and outline, see Annas and Grodin (2008, 136f). The historical origins go back to the Nuremberg trial after the Second World War. Judges condemning the deeds of Nazi doctors during the Third Reich promulgated this legal and ethical code to avoid future atrocities regarding

experiments on humans. The Nuremberg Code is a primary foundational document informing all subsequent ethical codes on research involving human subjects. Many consider it the most authoritative legal and human rights code for experimentation with humans (Annas and Grodin 2008).

6 For a detailed introduction and outline, see Beauchamp (2008, 149f). In brief, the Belmont Report is an ethics document containing moral principles for research with humans, which was published in 1979 by the US National Commission for the Protection of Human Subjects of Biomedical and Behavioral Research (National Commission). The National Commission came into existence in 1974 after a public outrage and congressional uncertainty over the famous Tuskegee syphilis experiments. Here, African American men were enrolled in experiments and subject to ethically unjustifiable forms of manipulation by health professionals. Other reports of the abuse of prisoners, children, and the "mentally infirm" in medical experiments appeared at that time. Even though drafted in the research context of the United States, it has gained wide recognition in many other countries (Beauchamp 2008, 49).

7 For a detailed introduction and outline, see Ashcroft (2008, 141f). The Declaration of Helsinki, entitled World Medical Association Declaration of Helsinki: Ethical Principles for Medical Association, is an official policy document of the World Medical Association (WMA). The establishment of the WMA was almost contemporaneous with the Nuremberg doctors' trial, the establishment of the United Nations, and the adoption of the Universal Declaration of Human Rights (Ashcroft 2008, 141).

8 For a detailed introduction and outline, see Idämpään-Heikkilä and Fluss (2008, 168ff). The Council established by the two UN agencies, WHO and UNESCO, first proposed in 1982 the International Guidelines for Biomedical Research Involving Human Subjects to indicate how the ethical principles in the WMA's Declaration of Helsinki (note 12) could be effectively interpreted and applied given socioeconomic circumstances, laws, regulations, and institutional arrangements. Additionally, the CIOMS-WHO guidelines were thought to specifically address research ethics in LMIC contexts. The guidelines were effectively promulgated and revised in 1993, 2002, and 2016 (Idämpään-Heikkilä and Fluss 2008, 168).

9 The International Bioethics Committee (IBC) is a body of thirty-six independent experts created in 1993 that evaluates and follows progress in the life sciences and its applications to ensure respect for humans (UNESCO 2019).

10 Admittedly, "population" is also an ambiguous term, as in some contexts, a study population refers to the potential participants of a study defined by inclusion or exclusion criteria (for instance, children or female adults with certain health conditions).

11 The following text excerpt is a reconstruction of the "Havrix trial" drawn from Hawkins and Emanuel (2008, 55ff).

12 The purposes of Phase 2 trials are to evaluate the short-term safety of a drug, to confirm the clinical efficacy of a drug, and to determine the therapeutic dose range. Phase 3 tests the effectiveness of the treatment or cure of a specific condition; see Section "Global Health Research in Low-Income Communities: Setting the Stage."

13 The following case is drawn and summarized from Hawkins and Emanuel (2008, 1–2).

Chapter 2

1 The wording of the CIOMS-WHO guidelines (2016, paragraph 1) is as follows: "[T]he ethical justification of health-related research involving humans is its social value: the prospect of generating the knowledge and/or the means necessary to protect and promote people's health. Clinicians, researchers, policy makers, public health officials, patients, pharmaceutical companies, and others rely on the results of research for activities and decisions that impact individual and public health, welfare, and the use of limited resources. [...] Such research must always be carried out in ways that uphold human rights, and respect, protect, and are fair to study participants and the communities in which the research is conducted."

2 Wertheimer's theory has been widely applied to many topics in biomedical ethics and in the research ethics literature (Emanuel et al. 2008; Malmqvist and Szigeti 2021; Resnik 2003), even by Wertheimer himself (2011), and has been criticized, discussed, and expanded (London 2005, 2008; Macklin 2004; Malmqvist 2013; Mitra 2012; Snyder 2012; Wenner 2016). There is certainly a much richer tradition of theories of exploitation, including Marxist, libertarian, and Kantian accounts, to name but a few (e.g., Cohen 2008; Elster 1985; Ferguson and Zwolinski 2024; Goodin 1987; Reeve 1987; Roemer 1996; Sample 2003; Valdman 2008, 2009; Vrousalis 2013; Wood 1995; Young 2009, 2011).

3 For the conceptual specifications and exact argument, see Chapter 3.

4 For a good literature overview, see London (2012) on the social value requirement as a valuable principle that safeguards public trust (see also Holzer 2017). See Resnik (2016) for a critique.

Chapter 3

1 I shall note that the vulnerability model is not explicitly "transactional." However, obligations and fairness requirements are formulated as applying to "agreements" between researchers with their sponsors and communities, which I interpret as tantamount to transactions.

2 I shall clarify that there are other important normative models that rely on a nonpolitical "moral individualism," such as some cosmopolitan approaches. In Chapter 5, I will further discuss common cosmopolitan models applied to the context of international health research, such as the "human development approach" (London 2005, 2008), Pratt and Loff's (2013) "promotion of justice in global health through health research," and Pogge's (2002) global health reform scheme based on human rights. These cosmopolitan approaches deserve and will receive their own discussion, as they make an important contribution to global justice and more general obligations or duties toward the global poor.

3 There may be additional ethical requirements, e.g., an obligation to strengthen the capacity of host communities or collaborative partnerships between researchers (and their sponsors) and host countries (Pratt and Loff 2014). As I further explain, these requirements can be seen in the wider context of the economic model.

4 Wertheimer (2011, 277) discusses moral principles and justifications associated with the classical problems in research ethics in light of what he—alternatively—calls the "economic model" or the "contractual model." This model is thought to describe and analyze the normative relationships among researchers, sponsors, and research participants. I will use the term "economic model" to refer to the fair benefits approach. I shall note that there is a striking parallel between the framework developed by Wertheimer and that of Emanuel and colleagues: the fair benefit approach heavily draws on the principles and premises that Wertheimer introduces in the "economic model." In this sense, I contend that the "economic model" can be expanded to issues related to the fair treatment of host communities.

5 I would like to acknowledge that the concept of vulnerability is certainly equivocal and needs further clarification (for further reading, see Hurst 2008; Hurst 2020; Luna 2009, 2019; Martin and Hurst 2017). I cannot develop or outline a sound conceptualization of vulnerability without straying beyond my stated aims. However, as I will explain below, I adhere to the intuitive notion that individuals in precarious economic and health situations are vulnerable in the sense that they are prone to agree to exploitative offers (or are less able to reject unethical research proposals).

6 Here, I will summarize different interpretations of both requirements under the label "vulnerability model." To do this, I will ignore interpretive conflicts and rival conceptualizations of responsiveness and reasonable availability.

7 See previous note 56, Luna (2009, 2019), Hurst (2008), and Martin and Hurst (2017).

8 In Section "Three Objections against Transactional Models for Fair Benefit-sharing," I will furthermore explain that both accounts, the economic and the vulnerability model, fail to offer a sound conception of (community) exploitation.

9 Equipoise is defined as a state in which there is insufficient evidence to warrant a judgment that one intervention in the trial is superior or inferior to the others.

10 I leave a more detailed discussion of the problem of "undue inducement" in health research to Chapter 8.

11 I specify and discuss the principles of collaborative partnership and transparency in Section 'Mechanisms' in Chapter 7.

12 Note that in the literature, the exploiter is usually reconstructed as A and the exploited party as B. Gbadegesin and Wendler (2006) reconstruct the case in the opposite way: B is the exploiter and A the exploited.

13 The "basic structure" of society (Rawls TJ, sect. 2) is the design of the basic social and political institutions that structure daily life and individuals' decisions and actions, and which distribute fundamental rights and duties and determine the division of advantages of social cooperation. According to Rawls, the basic structure of society is the "first subject" of justice, as it has a profound impact on character formation and the life prospects of people and is necessary for background justice. The principles of justice apply directly to the basic institutions, comprising the political constitution, the legal system of trials,

property, contracts, the system of markets, the regulation of economic relations, and the family (Freeman 2007, 464).

14 As Arneson (2016, 17f) notes, the fact that I have no power to alter the terms of interaction in my favor on a fully competitive market does not mean that my transaction with others, by taking advantage of competitive conditions, is always fair. Moreover, he argues that the equilibrium on a fully competitive (Pareto-optimal) market is at most a minimal condition of fairness, but not more than that (Arneson 2016, 18).

15 There may be additional arguments to show that a free market constitutes a moral institution that contributes to social cohesion, solidarity, and integration of individuals (Markovits 2017).

16 I already presented some of the following critiques in the previous chapter. Here, I want to offer the conceptual underpinnings for these objections.

17 One should note that Millum's (2011) examples and Wertheimer's account align with anarchist authors such as Nozick (1974), Simmons (1979a, 2001) who refuse to accept prima facie obligations across agent networks in cooperative schemes. Obligations are a priori invalid, as they violate agents' autonomy (Dagger and Lefkowitz 2014). That is, if I do not voluntarily join a community, I do not have the moral obligation to pay taxes in order to pay a community worker's salary. Other scholars have argued for the weaker, a posteriori thesis that existing theories of obligations have failed to make the case that individual agents are obligations-bearers who owe these obligations to institutions and the community as a whole (Dagger and Lefkowitz 2014; Simmons 1979b, 2001, chap. 6). On these views, the moral ground of obligations should be associated with transaction-specific fairness obligations that arise between individual agents.

18 Any specific moral claim(-right) on benefits must be matched by some corresponding obligation, which is assigned to an obligation-bearer (O'Neill 1996).

19 As an important side note, it needs to be mentioned that Wertheimer (2011, 258) even rejects the postulation of special obligations that emerge from direct interactions if framed as obligations to provide super-contractual benefits. He says, referring to the fair benefits approach: "Although some of the claims as to what researchers should do for participants or their communities can be couched in the procrustean bed of avoiding exploitation, the force of IP [the emergence of super-contractual obligations on the basis of interactions] goes beyond what can sensibly be put in those terms and deserves a more thorough

and focused discussion" (Wertheimer 2011, 256, edited). Obligations to provide super-contractual obligations are obligations to provide additional benefits that the interacting parties do not agree upon in their contract. It can be objected that super-contractual obligations are often merely contractual if A interacts with B knowing that she acquires obligations that go beyond those to which A and B would otherwise have agreed. For instance, A may know that she owes B the minimum wage even though they agreed to a wage under the minimum level—but A does not owe more than this (e.g., benefits beyond the minimum wage) (Wertheimer 2011, 259). Wertheimer is right in claiming that obligations cannot be super-contractual in this sense. But I cannot see why this would be a general objection to special obligations, as Wertheimer seems to assume (Wertheimer 2011, 256). I interpret special obligations as contractual obligations that reflect fair transaction terms. Fair benefits are benefits that are owed to another party acquired through an interaction. This does not necessarily imply that those benefits are super-contractual.

20 To make a clarifying point, Hughes' (2014) argument is built upon special obligations, not exploitation. However, both concepts are closely related in a micro-fairness account. The argument goes that if there are no transaction-specific obligations, the situation is not prone to exploitation because without obligations of fairness arising from a transaction, unfair advantage cannot be taken.

21 Chapter 6 will deepen the conceptual connection between structural injustice and transaction-specific exploitation.

22 This idea shows similarity to Nozick's (1974) account, on which an existing holding will be just if it arises from an act of just initial acquisition followed by one or more acts of just transfer. A just transfer is characterized by its just terms.

23 I only reconstruct the core of the argument London and Zollman (2010) develop throughout their paper. The overall economic analysis is much more complex.

Chapter 4

1 This symmetry between a fair distribution and (non)exploitation follows to a certain extent the approach Wertheimer (1999) defends: exploitation is defined as the noncompliance with a fairness constraint.

2 As explained in the introduction (Chapter 1), I am using the classification of "special (perfect) obligations" (owed to a specific body of agents) and "universal (perfect) duties" (owed to everyone) (see O'Neill's 1996, 152).

3 However, there might be other options left to ground special obligations in joint agency. For instance, Bratman (1999) relies on additional morally binding promises or contracts that are often present in joint enterprises (Alonso 2008, 89).

4 See Chapter 3, and explanation in Section "Basic Structures—a Solution?," Chapter 4.

5 I will use both terms synonymously.

6 I acknowledge that there are many different interpretations of the principle of fairness; I do not have space here to discuss them all.

7 According to Hart, "[t]he rules may provide that officials should have authority to enforce obedience and make further rules, and this will create a structure of legal rights and duties, but the moral obligation to obey the rules in such circumstances is due to the cooperating members of the society" (Hart 1955, 185).

8 According to Simmons (1979a, 317), even if we can agree that intolerably unjust schemes ought not to be furthered, there is no logical difficulty, at least, in holding that we have obligations of fairness to cooperate within "moderately" unjust schemes. Here, it can also be argued that especially the most privileged beneficiaries have at least prima facie obligations to reciprocate their fair contribution to others in a collaborative scheme.

9 To make the point clear, consider the following example: people decide to install a public entertainment system with music, funny stories and so forth provided in a public space. Some people living in the neighborhood may happen to open the window occasionally and listen to the music or chuckle at a funny story (Nozick 1974, 95). According to Nozick's (1974) view, people who occasionally open the windows (without intention of listening to the entertainment) are not morally required to contribute to the public entertainment scheme, even if they receive benefits. I here follow Nozick, arguing that individuals who unintentionally happen to receive benefits do not necessarily bear fairness obligations.

10 This relies on Kutz's (2000, 100) distinction between intended and intentional action. He argues that "individuals can intentionally contribute to a collective end even though they do not intend the realization of that end." In other words, "agents who intentionally perform their part of some joint end, but who lack a

group-intention of realizing that joint act, nonetheless intentionally perform an act as a means to the joint end" (Kutz 2000, 100).

11 Again, free-rider conduct can only be morally worrisome if the cause of a benefit-creating activity is just. Members of the Camorra may "free-ride" on the positive effects of a murder of one of their enemies, committed by one of their fellows. Dworkin (2011, 315) thinks, however, that this cannot build a basis for the moral condemnation of free-riders, given that no (moral) obligations can be imposed on cooperators of a scheme lacking a just end.

12 This is also in line with Chauvier's (2013, 199) definition: free-riding by a party B on another party A's efforts occurs if B recurrently and continuously uses something A produces or has produced, and either reduces the value and utility available for A, or does not contribute (with her own efforts or resources) to A's production.

13 One may object that from a self-interested perspective, some community members, like the healthy ones, always contribute disproportionately more than they benefit from a working health system compared to the ill and needy. The point is, however, that socially valuable knowledge in order to be considered truly socially valuable for a community only needs to be potentially transformable into a health benefit that accrues to a representative cross-section of potential future patients in the community.

14 To avoid confusion, note that Wenner (2018a) originally develops her model to ground the "social value requirement" in health research. I, however, focus on obligations of fair benefit-sharing.

15 Wenner (2019) justifiably objects to the previous argument that there are "relational" cosmopolitans who argue that the principles of (distributive) justice in Rawls extend to the global sphere. For instance Beitz (1979, 1983) and Pogge (2002, 2005a) have argued that there exist interactions between international agents regulated by international institutions and that these transactions not only give rise to a duty of justice, i.e., to create and maintain just international institutions but also to a global application of principles of distributive justice. Without further investigating this approach at this point, I would like to emphasize one possible worry: I do not think that cosmopolitan accounts can show that researchers and sponsors participate in a collaborative scheme with a specific host community and thus bear special obligations, as the relational scheme they present is of global extent and not country- or community-specific. I will deepen this argument in Chapter 5.

16 For a detailed account of beneficiaries, benefit-creating schemes, and the ethics of benefiting, see also Chauvier (2013, chap. 5).

17 Here, it should be noted that is widely considered true that intellectual property protections are necessary for companies to initiate research projects at all (Lester 2016).

18 I shall note that it is not always obvious that such burdens (typical of well-ordered states where public goods are financed by tax payments) can easily be applied to extremely deprived low-income countries. The public goods, if they exist, are frequently financed by the rent on natural resources and by external public aid. So, tax contributions are only one form of relevant restriction.

19 This conception of community is endogenous and relative to the theory of stakeholder fairness. I acknowledge that, e.g., Rawls distinguishes community—a unity of people following a shared comprehensive doctrine—from well-ordered societies that leave room for reasonable pluralism (Rawls PL, 40).

20 Since I still owe an account for background injustices, I will address the non-ideal structural context and its conceptual connection to community exploitation in more detail in Chapter 6. I will argue that non-ideal circumstances are explanatory for community exploitation because the relative frequency of community exploitation is increased in unjust circumstances.

21 Chapter 7 further specifies the scope and kinds of benefits under the fair play model.

22 In a more recent paper, Klosko (2014) states that individuals may reject essential goods under some circumstances. Klosko (2014, 164) admits that people can refuse to cooperate in the case of (even nonexcludable) essential goods on grounds of a strong desire to reject the good in question, if reasonable arguments are provided. So, he concedes that a minimum level of participatory intentions must be given to place individuals under obligations. Nevertheless, refusing to cooperate, especially in the case of nonexcludable goods, such as tax payments for national defense, is very difficult. This is owed to the following problem: to figure out whether individuals have intentions to free-ride on a provided benefit or good reasons to refuse contribution to a good poses extreme epistemic hurdles in real life (Klosko 2014, 168). The question is whether, for instance, a pacifist can legitimately refuse to pay taxes for national defense on the ground of her beliefs.

23 Libertarians, such as Nozick and Simmons, would probably just deny this, claiming that voluntary consent is at the heart of obligation. Also, Rehfeld

(2005, 420) casts doubt on whether Klosko (1992, 2005) is able to ground obligations on the fact that a good is presumptively necessary. Nevertheless, he argues that Klosko's account could be broadened, arguing that everyone has an obligation to preserve her own life. By analogy, this account can be based on other accounts requiring individuals to abandon the state of nature, such as theories by Hobbes, Locke, or Kant.

24 Klosko's (2005, 2014) account focuses for the most part on essential public goods. So, if we develop his argument further, we probably need to adhere to a conceptualization of health research as contributing to essential public benefits. I will not enter the discussion about whether health is a public or private good. However, I acknowledge that this discussion would be useful in order to strengthen Klosko's (2005, 34) suggestion that health research contributes to and fosters public health (as an essential public good).

25 We may wonder if nonpayment on the part of beneficiaries displays a blameworthy moral attitude, independently of obligations under a theory of fair play. For instance, Chauvier (2013, 204) suggests that each beneficiary of a beneficial scheme should adopt a constant concern ("inquiétude") to pay: "you ought to be concerned to know whether the external beneficial effects of the activities of others should be paid (Tu dois t'inquiéter de savoir si les effets externes bénéfiques des activités des autres ne sont pas payants)."

26 For more details see Dagger and Lefkowitz (2014).

Chapter 5

1 Sen (1993, 1999) has drawn a lot of attention to the capability approach for the evaluation of public policies. Here, he opposes to the Rawlsian focus on primary goods and argues that the capability approach captures the different effects of the same bundle of goods on different people (Ruger 2009, 53).

2 See also London and Kimmelman's version: "protocols [should] be defined as responsive to the health needs of the host community only if they are part of a programme of inquiry that will expand the capacity of health-related social structures in the host community to meet urgent health needs" (2008, 82).

3 It should be clarified that a human right to *X* (e.g., health) does not mean that an agent has necessarily the right to access a particular health intervention. The scope and extent of *X* has to be defined by institutions (see also Daniels 2015).

4 While a positive duty puts an obligation to do an act on the person on whom it is imposed, a negative duty implies forbearance on the part of the person on whom it is imposed.

5 For a more comprehensive overview of Pogge's framework and of the most prominent critique, see Sonderholm (2012): "Thomas Pogge on Global Justice and World Poverty: A Review Essay."

6 Even though this is not the case for all essential medicines, as some of them are not under patent protection (Jha et al. 2002).

7 However, Pogge (2008) discusses the non-ideal case in which mutually beneficial research under a double standard (see Chapter 2) is presumably unethical. Under the assumption that a double standard leads to more mutually advantageous clinical trials in developing nations (as sponsors tend to outsource trials under a double standard to LMICs), we cannot give a unique response to the question whether a double standard is morally legitimate. This is the case because research subjects receive benefits, even if those benefits are insufficient under a double standard. I will raise this non-ideal point in more detail in the final discussion (Chapter 8).

8 Pogge insists on perfect (negative) duties with corresponding rights-holders. Regarding the duty to aid in London's (2005) account, we can also argue that this duty is perfect, given that if an agent is in the right position, she has a perfect duty to help the needy. Also, I would like to emphasize that London (2005) seems to proceed from a counterpart "right" held by the needy whose human flourishing is central. Here, the needy have claims to be helped. Pratt and Loff (2014) argue similar things. In contrast, O'Neill's (1996) duty of virtue and Millum's (2011) duty of beneficence take the duty-bearer as a starting point, not the rights-claimer.

9 Importantly, Millum (2011) addresses obligations to research subjects and not host community members. However, his argument can easily be transferred to communities, as general duties of beneficence do not only apply to a specific class of people, such as research subjects.

10 The fair play model does not compete with cosmopolitan theories in the sense that both can be correct. However, special obligations under the fair play model and universal cosmopolitan duties might generate conflicts if they cannot be discharged at the same time, given that resources are limited.

11 Similar to the terminology applied in Chapter 4, I will use the "principle of fair play" and the "principle of stakeholder fairness" (as outlined by Phillips [1997]) as synonyms.

12 The European Medicines Agency (EMA 2019) lists Havrix as an approved vaccine in Europe. Similarly, the Paul Ehrlich Institute (2019), a German research institution and medical regulatory body, and the German Federal Institute for Vaccines and Biomedicines state that companies, such as GlaxoSmithKline, CC Pharma, or EurimPharm, hold sub-licenses of the Havrix vaccine.

13 For the sake of the argument, I assume that A does not benefit from global public health; or global public health benefits generated in other countries can at least be neglected.

14 I am adhering to Barry's use of the term "fair play."

15 For instance, I previously argued that traders are obliged to pay fair prices for the goods they buy. However, this does not imply a fairness obligation to share benefits with the global poor beyond that (Chapter 4).

16 Phillips' (1997) principle of stakeholder fairness is based on the assumption that the acceptance of (any kind of) benefit in a mutually beneficial (and just) cooperative scheme (as opposed to transactions) places an agent under fairness obligations.

17 Public goods can be subdivided into pure public goods where every individual necessarily consumes the same unit of the good (e.g., national defense) and collective goods where individuals do not necessarily consume the same amount of a good (e.g., a TV broadcast signal that can only be received by a special device) (Arneson 1982, 619).

18 We may need to add complexity to the public goods account: strictly speaking, agents cannot accept benefits resulting from pure public goods. This is the case because nobody can be excluded from them. There may be some public benefits resulting from what I call quasi-collective knowledge. For instance, some people may benefit from national security due to the use of new vaccines in the military (see the Havrix case).

Chapter 6

1 As I explained in Chapter 3, structural or "background injustices" subsume a wide range of structural factors—including a lack of education, insufficient access to health care, political and economic instability, or distributive inequalities (Malmqivst 2013, 560)—that are deemed to be striking features of research settings in LMICs.

2 The case description is verbatim from Malmqvist (2013).

3 In Section "Mapping Competing Accounts of Exploitation," I will offer a more specific overview of common transaction-specific accounts of exploitation.

4 Here, I follow Wood's (1995) claim that any conception of exploitation always points at a morally wrong relationship between two parties A and B. This account is opposed to interpretations of exploitation that treat it as morally neutral (see Feinberg 1989).

5 This reconstruction is based on the manuscript Exploitation and Joint Action by Malmqvist and Szigeti (2019). Furthermore, I would like to emphasize that, although listed among purely transactional accounts, some authors do not preclude the structural viewpoint: e.g., Snyder (2012) and Sample (2003) are not only committed to the transaction-specific account but also acknowledge the structural interpretation of exploitation.

6 Malmqvist (2013) draws on Kutz's (2000) account of complicity developed for the context of organized collective actions. An accomplice bears a relation to some collectively caused harm by virtue of which she is accountable for that harm (Malmqvist 2013, 568).

7 See also the cases Rescuer or Ant and Grasshopper in Vrousalis (2013, 148–50).

8 My strategy is to accept cases like Antidote as exploitation. Roemer would probably contest this claim and say that Antidote relates to a moral wrong other than exploitation, as the case is not the immediate consequence of (distributive) injustice. My rationale is that this chapter aims to show that even if we accept the purely transaction-specific view, we ought to account for the structural concerns.

9 The relative frequency of an event $Z \in \Omega$ is defined as the number of times that the event occurs in a specified context divided by the total number of events Ω.

10 For a detailed overview of theories of probabilistic causation, see Hitchcock (2018). Causation as referring to significant correlations is still in line with what Hart and Honoré (1985) have called the common sense understanding of causation. According to this understanding, we say that C causes E when we single out C as one among a potentially large number of antecedent conditions for E's occurrence, distinguished from other conditions by virtue of its abnormality.

11 To clarify: I only use the example as an analogy to make clear the causal-explanatory relationship between two concepts (or variables).

12 Pearl (2000) has challenged the probabilistic theory of causation. He argues that the conditional probability $P(E| C)$ represents a probability resulting form

a passive observation of an event C. Indeed, observing the barometer falling increases the probability of a storm coming, but does not "cause" the storm. Consequently, Reichenbach (1956) has argued that if neither A nor B is a cause of the other, but A and B are correlated variables, there must be always a common cause C that causally explains the correlation between A and B. In this regard, we may accept the causal thesis underlying "probability raising."

13 At this point, I would like to mention that in the exploitation case, an inverse causal relationship is possible, namely, that exploitation causes or enables unjust structures to persist.

14 My use of the term "systemic" is to distinguish a subset of transactional exploitation that I consider to be causally linked to background injustice. This should not be confused with other uses of the term "systemic" in the literature, such as "structural-systemic," which is one of three heuristic categories that explain how structural injustice is reproduced (Wiedenbrug 2018).

15 Here, I leave aside the view by egalitarians, such as Wolff (1998) or Rawls (TJ), who argue that taking the egalitarian project seriously means that egalitarian principles of justice should contribute to the formation of people with egalitarian characters that act reciprocally. In this sense, there could be considerably fewer non-systemic exploitative actions in just egalitarian societies, as people's characters are forged by mutual respect and equal concern. I am aware of this argument, but I think that it does not conceptually invalidate the distinction between systemic and non-systemic exploitation.

16 Note that there can also be unjust contexts in HICs, for instance, in low-income contexts in which some individuals are significantly worse-off than others (CIOMS-WHO 2016, guideline 2). For instance, in the political and economic realities of life in states like the United States, access to health care and economic security are not assured for all people. Thus, enrollment in clinical trials can serve as an incentive for relatively disadvantaged people to access care or income (Fisher 2009, 161–2; see Kolata and Eichenwald 1999). Nevertheless, we may generally observe that (especially severe) background injustices prevail in LMICs.

17 Again, I am interested in the conceptual relationship of different variables and do not pretend to use the smoking analogy as a normative example of structural injustice.

18 Wilson (2009) argues (regarding normative frameworks) that the factors of complex systems can make the application of moral arguments from simplistic top-down approaches invalid.

19 For a comprehensive multi-principled "connection theory" of remedial responsibilities grounded in causal, moral, capacity, and community based considerations, see Miller (2001a).

20 The interested reader will also find an in-depth analysis of the topic in work by Eduardo Rivera-Lopez (2017).

21 Malmqvist (2017, 485) himself does not explicitly take position regarding the prohibition of exploitative trials.

Chapter 7

1 For an outline of the difference principle, see Section "The Difference Principle Applied to Health Research."

2 For now, let me note that, for reasons of simplicity, I will discuss "principles of distributive justice" to identify valuable criteria for determining a fair distribution of benefits and burdens in a cooperative scheme. I here deliberately abstract from their application to formal institutions and basic structures.

3 Remember that I explained in Chapter 3, following London and Zollman (2010), that communities are frequently not sufficiently empowered to negotiate on equal terms. This is based on the assumption that researchers and sponsors hold "monopolies" on the market where highly desirable research projects are "sold" to potential host LMICs.

4 For a good overview of mechanisms, see Pratt (2021), who discusses her health equity framework in the light of global health research mechanisms for equitable benefit-sharing.

5 In Chapter 8, I will discuss a major problem associated with the appropriateness of benefits, namely, what is commonly known as "undue inducement." This is tantamount to an offer of excessive, unwarranted or inappropriate benefits to obtain consent for high-risk studies (National Commission 1979).

6 Remember that the responsiveness and reasonable availability requirements are necessary, but not sufficient moral demands. Additional benefits may be provided to the host communities (Chapter 3).

7 Rawls (TJ, TJR) conceives of society as a cooperative scheme. Distributive justice, for Rawls, applies to individuals that have a prior claim on the produced goods in question in virtue of cooperating to produce them. Allocative justice, in turn, applies when a given collection of goods is to be divided among definite

individuals with known desires and needs (Rawls 1971, 77). In circumstances of allocative justice, certain information about the parties to whom goods are to be allocated is given; and most importantly, the goods are not the product of individuals' cooperation, which means that people have no "prior" claims on the goods to be distributed (Murray 2015). Allocative justice applies on the basis of need and not cooperation.

8 For a comprehensive overview of distributive principles outside the health context, see Lamont (2017a,b).

9 See note 148.

10 Rawls further used the maximin decision rule to argue that parties in the original position would choose his principles of justice. First, he shows that maximin is an appropriate decision rule, requiring choosers to select the option whose worst outcome is better than the worst outcomes of each of the other options. Rawls then argues that if the parties in the original position employed the maximin rule, they would choose Rawls' principles of justice (Rawls TJ, 150ff; Lamont 2017b).

11 I argued in Chapter 6 that background injustices make community exploitation more likely. But this rather justifies emphasizing and assigning remedial responsibilities to actors who then ought to remedy background injustices.

12 However, admittedly, an improved version (not applied to single interactions) of the difference principle would ask from an international research institution to collect tax money from all research interactions in order to redistribute this money according to the difference principle. Here, Ballantyne would also owe an account of how tax money would be collected and redistributed.

13 Accountability for reasonableness has been employed as a guide to policymaking in multiple situations, notably including the efforts of the Mexican government and the World Health Organization to tackle HIV/AIDS in LMICs. Daniels' model has also had a great influence on the British National Health Service and the National Institute for Health and Care Excellence (Badano 2014).

14 Accountability for reasonableness is an account tailored to allocative justice, see note 149.

15 For an in-depth critique of the four conditions constituting accountability for reasonableness, notably the relevance condition, see Friedman (2008). I abstain from critically discussing Daniels and Sabin's conditions here, as the aim of the chapter is to outline an alternative to the currently accepted frameworks that

present either end-state or procedural market accounts to achieve fair benefit-sharing.

16 As Daniels (2000) explains, in pluralist social contexts, we find reasonable disagreement about principles that should govern priority-setting: some may give more priority to the worst off, some less, and some want to aggregate benefits in ways that others do not.

17 Meckled-Garcia (2013) addresses the context of institutionalizing social and economic human rights.

18 Yet, as Jha (2002) convincingly shows, there are also huge health deficits and inequities related to the lack of basic medicines that are not affected by patents.

Chapter 8

1 I would like to acknowledge the importance of the basic structure and cosmopolitan models. Nevertheless, my discussion will focus on the two predominant transactional models, which is owed to stipulations with the scope of my final chapter and also because my primary critique containing three fundamental objections was directed toward these transactional models.

2 It is certainly worth noting that I have also addressed the ethics of individual research subjects, in particular in Chapters 2 and 6.

3 As Malmqvist (2017, 478) argues, if we hold that the non-worseness claim is true, we may, as a first option, accept that neglect is much worse than we thought and exploitation should no longer be condemned, which would result in a relaxation of ethical standards. As a second option, we may, however, claim that ethical standards should be strengthened and sponsors are placed under a duty to conduct non-exploitative trials in LMICs. In both cases, neglect (no clinical trials) remains indefensible.

4 Of course, this does not exclude that non-ideal circumstances can be acknowledged as factors that complicate the achievement of a fairness norm (Chapter 6).

5 Emanuel (2004) here refers to research subjects and not communities.

Bibliography

Access to Medicines Foundation. "Commentary: Edging Closer to Lenacapavir Access in Low- and Middle-Income Countries." 2025. https://accesstomedicinefoundation.org/access-insights/commentary-edging-closer-to-lenacapavir-access-in-low-and-middle-income-countries.

African Union & Africa CDC. "Launch of Partnerships for African Vaccine Manufacturing (PAVM)." 2021. https://africacdc.org/wp-content/uploads/2021/04/post-summit-comunique-African-Union-and-Africa-CDC-launches-Partnerships-for-African-Vaccine-Manufacturing.pdf.

Albertsen, Andreas. "A Vaccine Tax: Ensuring a More Equitable Global Vaccine Distribution." *Journal of Medical Ethics* 48, no. 10 (2022): 658–61.

Alonso, Facundo. "Shared Intention, Reliance, and Interpersonal Obligations: an Inquiry into the Metaphysics and Interpersonal Normativity of Shared Agency." PhD thesis, 2008, available at https://searchworks.stanford.edu/view/7915317 [accessed March 13, 2026].

Alves, Lise. "Brazil to Start Widespread Dengue Vaccinations." *The Lancet* 403, no. 10387 (2024): 133.

Amri, M., J. Filart, and Jesse B. Bump. "The Quest for Equity in Global Health Is Underpinned by Neocolonial Discourses: A Critical Discourse Analysis." *PLOS Global Public Health* 5, no. 6 (2025): e0004663.

Amri, Michelle, Jan Filart, Jinny Yang, Johanna Manga, Kathryn Barrett, and Jesse B. Bump. "Decolonizing Global Health: A Scoping Review of Its Key Components, Proposed Actions, and Contributors." *Global Health Research and Policy* 10, no. 1 (2025): 54.

Andanda, Pamela, Doris Schroeder, Sachin Chaturvedi, Emezat Mengesha, and Tim Hodges. "Legal Frameworks for Benefit Sharing: From Biodiversity to Human Genomics." In *Benefit Sharing: From Biodiversity to Human Genetics*, edited by D. Schroeder and J. Cook Lucas, 33–64. Dordrecht: Springer, 2013.

Angell, Marcia. "Ethical Imperialism? Ethics in International Collaborative Clinical Research." *The New England Journal of Medicine* 319, no. 16 (1988): 1081–3.

Angell, Marcia. "The Ethics of Clinical Research in the Third World." *The New England Journal of Medicine* 337, no. 12 (1997): 847–9.

Annas, George J., and Michael A. Grodin. "Human Rights and Maternal-Fetal HIV Transmission Prevention Trials in Africa." *American Journal of Public Health* 88, no. 4 (1998): 560–3.

Annas, George J., and Michael A. Grodin. "The Nuremberg Code." In *The Oxford Textbook of Clinical Research Ethics*, edited by E. J. Emanuel et al., 136–40. Oxford: Oxford University Press, 2008.

Appiah, Kwame Anthony. *Cosmopolitanism: Ethics in a World of Strangers*. New York: W. W. Norton, 2006.

Arendt, Hannah. "Collective Responsibility." In *Amor Mundi: Explorations in the Faith and Thought of Hannah Arendt*, edited by J. W. Bernauer, 43–50. Boston, MA: M. Nijhoff, 1987.

Arneson, Richard. "Broadly Utilitarian Theories of Exploitation and Multinational Clinical Research." In *Exploitation and Developing Countries: The Ethics of Clinical Research*, edited by J. S. Hawkins and E. J. Emanuel, 286–313. Princeton, NJ: Princeton University Press, 2008.

Arneson, Richard. "Exploitation, Domination, Competitive Markets, and Unfair Division." *The Southern Journal of Philosophy* 54, Spindel Supplement (2016): 9–30. https://onlinelibrary.wiley.com/doi/pdf/10.1111/sjp.12182?casa_token=g4zs2tJawPEAAAAA%3AEoNEwFvMtamu4htVcyhUf2tpT5dl28cpse59QanBTmRA3KIu9JNOmA1U-aBHUz3eeXYMzorZjiYQHA

Arneson, Richard J. "The Principle of Fairness and Free-Rider Problems." *Ethics* 92, no. 4 (1982): 616–33.

Aristotle. *Nicomachean Ethics*. Translated by R. Bartlett and S. D. Collins. Chicago, IL: University of Chicago Press, 2011.

Ashcroft, Richard. "The Declaration of Helsinki." In *The Oxford Textbook of Clinical Research Ethics*, edited by E. J. Emanuel et al., 141–8. Oxford: Oxford University Press, 2008.

Azariadis, Costas, and Stachurski John. "Poverty Traps." In *Handbook of Economic Growth*, edited by P. Aghion and S. N. Durlauf, Vol. 1, 295–384. Amsterdam: Elsevier, 2005.

Badano, Garbiele. "Deliberative Democracy, Public Reason and the Allocation of Clinical Care Resources." PhD thesis, 2014, available at http://discovery.ucl.ac.uk/1453168/.

Ballantyne, Angela J. "HIV International Clinical Research: Exploitation and Risk." *Bioethics* 19, no. 5-6 (2005): 476–91.

Ballantyne, Angela J. "Benefits to Research Subjects in International Trials: Do They Reduce Exploitation or Increase Undue Inducement?" *Developing World Bioethics* 8, no. 3 (2008): 178–91.

Ballantyne, Angela J. "How to Do Research Fairly in an Unjust World." *The American Journal of Bioethics* 10, no. 6 (2010a): 26–35.

Ballantyne, Angela J. "Response to Open Peer Commentaries on 'How to Do Research Fairly in an Unjust World.'" *The American Journal of Bioethics* 10, no. 6 (2010b): W4–W6.

Banerjee, Amitava, Hollis, Aidan, et Pogge, Thomas. "The Health Impact Fund: Incentives for Improving Access to Medicines." *The Lancet* 375, no. 9709 (2010): 166–9.

Barry, Brian. "Humanity and Justice in Global Perspective." *NOMOS: Am. Soc'y Pol. Legal Phil.* 24 (1982): 219–52. https://www.jstor.org/stable/24219453

Barry, Christian et Wiens, David. "Benefiting from Wrongdoing and Sustaining Wrongful Harm." *Journal of Moral Philosophy* 13, no. 5 (2016): 530–52.

Barry, Michele. "Ethical Considerations of Human Investigation in Developing Countries." *The New England Journal of Medicine* 319, no. 16 (1988): 1083–6.

Barsdorf, Nicola et Millum, Joseph. "The Social Value of Health Research and the Worst Off." *Bioethics* 31, no. 2 (2017): 105–15.

Barugahare, John. "Can Resource-Poor Countries Bear Any Obligations for Global Distributive Justice? A Reflection on the Distribution of Global Health Opportunities." PhD thesis, 2016, available at https://nva.sikt.no/registration/0198cc3ca10b-ea55ca64-b59a-4ea5-9f6c-2861dc376859 [accessed April 4, 2026].

Barugahare, John et Lie, Reidar K. "Obligations of Poor Countries in Ensuring Global Justice: The Case of Uganda." *Etikk i praksis-Nordic Journal of Applied Ethics*, no. 2 (2014): 82–96.

Barugahare, John et Lie, Reidar K. "Obligations of Low Income Countries in Ensuring Equity in Global Health Financing." *BMC Medical Ethics* 16, no. 1 (2015): 59.

Basu, Jayasree. "Research on Disparities in Primary Health Care in Rural Versus Urban Areas: Select Perspectives." *International Journal of Environmental Research and Public Health* 19, no. 12 (2022): 7110.

Beauchamp, Tom L. "The Belmont Report." In *The Oxford Textbook of Clinical Research Ethics*, edited by E. J. Emanuel et al., 149–55. Oxford: Oxford University Press, 2008.

Beauchamp, Tom L., and James F. Childress. *Principles of Biomedical Ethics*. New York: Oxford University Press, 2001.

Beauchamp, Tom L., and James F. Childress. *Principles of Biomedical Ethics*. 6th ed. New York: Oxford University Press, 2009.

Beitz, Charles. *Political Theory and International Relations*. Princeton, NJ: Princeton University Press, 1979.

Beitz, Charles R. "Cosmopolitan Ideals and National Sentiment." *The Journal of Philosophy* 80, no. 10 (1983): 591–600.

Bharat Biotech. "Bharat Biotech's COVAXIN Phase III Data Published in The Lancet." Press release, November 12, 2021. https://www.bharat-biotech.com/images/press/bharat-biotech-covaxin-phase3-lancet-pressrelease.pdf?utm_source=chatgpt.com.

Blake, Michael. "Distributive Justice, State Coercion, and Autonomy." *Philosophy & Public Affairs* 30, no. 3 (2001): 257–96.

Bratman, Michael. *Faces of Intention: Selected Essays on Intention and Agency*. Cambridge: Cambridge University Press, 1999.

Bratman, Michael. *Shared Agency: A Planning Theory of Acting Together*. Oxford: Oxford University Press, 2014.

Brem, Jeremias, Bavatharani Elankeswaran, David Erne, Nadja Hedrich, Thibault Lovey, Viviana Marzetta, Laura Tarrago Salvado, Céline Züger, and Patricia Schlagenhauf. "Dengue 'Homegrown' in Europe (2022 to 2023)." *New Microbes and New Infections* 56 (2024): 101205.

Brigido, Rodrigo E. S. *Groups, Rules and Legal Practice*. Vol. 89. Berlin: Springer Science & Business Media, 2010.

Buchanan, Allen, Tony Cole, and Robert O. Keohane. "Justice in the Diffusion of Innovation." *Journal of Political Philosophy* 19, no. 3 (2011): 306–32.

Buchanan, Allen, Tony Cole, and Robert O. Keohane. "Justice in the Diffusion of Innovation." In *Political Theory Without Borders*, edited by Robert E. Goodin and James S. Fishkin, 133–61. Malden, MA: Wiley Blackwell, 2015.

Business Standard. "Zydus Cadila's COVID Vaccine ZyCoV-D to Be Used in Seven States Initially." November 20, 2021. https://www.business-standard.com/article/current-affairs/zydus-cadila-s-covid-vaccine-zycov-d-to-be-used-in-seven-states-initially-121120200804_1.html?utm_source=chatgpt.com.

Caballero Anthony, Mely. "Health and Human Security Challenges in Asia: New Agendas for Strengthening Regional Health Governance." *Australian Journal of International Affairs* 72, no. 6 (2018): 602–16.

Carse, Alisa L., and Margaret Olivia Little. "Exploitation and the Enterprise of Medical Research." In *Exploitation and Developing Countries: The Ethics of Clinical Research*, edited by J. S. Hawkins and E. J. Emanuel, 206–45. Princeton, NJ: Princeton University Press, 2008.

Cartwright, Nancy. "Causal Laws and Effective Strategies." *Nous* 13, no. 4 (1979): 419–37.

Centers for Disease Control and Prevention. "CDC Studies of AZT to Prevent Mother-to-Child HIV Transmission in Developing Countries." 1997. https://aidsinfo.nih.gov/news/363/cdc-studies-of-azt-to-prevent-mother-to-child-hiv-transmission-in-developing-countries.

Chapman, Nick, Anna Doubell, and Lisette Oversteegen. "Closing the Health Innovation Gap: Progress on Neglected Diseases." *The Lancet Global Health* 9, no. 10 (2021): e1354–5.

Charatan, Fred. "Surfactant Trial in Latin American Infants Criticised." *BMJ* 322, no. 7286 (2001): 575. https://www.ncbi.nlm.nih.gov/pmc/articles/PMC1119782/.

Chauvier, Stéphane. *Éthique Sans Visage. Le Problème des Effets Externes*. Paris: Librairie Philosophique J. Vrin, 2013.

Chen, Lincoln C., Tim G. Evans, and Richard A. Cash. "Health as a Global Public Good." In *Global Public Goods: International Cooperation in the 21st Century*, edited by I. Kaul, I. Grunberg, and M. Stern, 284–304. Oxford: Oxford University Press, 1999.

CIOMS-WHO. *International Guidelines for Biomedical Research Involving Human Subjects*. Geneva: Council for International Organizations of Medical Sciences, 1993.

CIOMS-WHO. *International Ethical Guidelines for Biomedical Research Involving Human Subjects*. Geneva: Council for International Organizations of Medical Sciences, 2002. https://globalhealthtrainingcentre.tghn.org/site_media/media/medialibrary/2011/04/CIOMS_International_Ethical_Guidelines_for_Biomedical_Research_Involving_Human_Subjects.pdf [accessed June 17, 2023].

CIOMS-WHO. *International Guidelines for Health-Related Research Involving Human Subjects*. Geneva: Council for International Organizations of Medical Sciences, 2016. http://www.cioms.ch/index.php/12-newsflash/400-cioms-inernational-ethical-guidelines.

Cohen, Gerald A. *History, Labour, and Freedom*. Oxford: Oxford University Press, 1988.

Cohen, Gerald A. "On the Currency of Egalitarian Justice." *Ethics* 99, no. 4 (1989): 906–44.

Cohen, Gerald A. *Self-Ownership, Freedom and Equality*. Cambridge: Cambridge University Press, 1995.

Cohen, Gerald A. *Rescuing Equality and Justice*. Cambridge, MA: Harvard University Press, 2008.

Cohen, Gerald A. *Why Not Socialism?* Princeton, NJ: Princeton University Press, 2009.

Cohen, Joshua. "Philosophy, Social Science, Global Poverty." In *Thomas Pogge and His Critics*, edited by A. Jaggar, 18–45. Cambridge: Polity Press, 2010.

Concannon, Thomas, Melissa Fuster, Tully Saunders, Kamal Patel, John B. Wong, Laurel K. Lesli, and Joseph Lau. "When and How Are We Engaging Stakeholders in Health Care Research?" *RAND Research Briefs*. 2015. https://www.rand.org/content/dam/rand/pubs/research_briefs/RB9800/RB9820/RAND_RB9820.pdf.

Consani, Cristina Foroni, Joel T. Klein, and Soraya Nour Sckell, eds. *Cosmopolitanism: From the Kantian Legacy to Contemporary Approaches*. Berlin: Duncker & Humblot, 2021.

Convention on Biological Diversity of the United Nations Environmental Programme (CBD). "The Convention on Biological Diversity (CBD)." 1992. https://www.cbd.int/doc/legal/cbd-en.pdf.

Cook, Chad, and Chris Sheets. "Clinical Equipoise and Personal Equipoise: Two Necessary Ingredients for Reducing Bias in Manual Therapy Trials." *Journal of Manual & Manipulative Therapy* 19, no. 1 (2011): 55–7.

Crouch, Robert A., and John D. Arras. "AZT Trials and Tribulations." *The Hastings Center Report* 28, no. 6 (1998): 26–34.

Cullity, Garrett. "Moral Free Riding." *Philosophy & Public Affairs* 24, no. 1 (1995): 3–34.

Dagger, Richard, and David Lefkowitz. "Political Obligation." *Stanford Encyclopedia of Philosophy*. 2014, available at https://plat.edu/entries/political-obligation/ [accessed February 4, 2026].

Dal-Ré, Rafael, Alex John London, Ezekiel Emanuel, and David Wendler. "The Potential Exploitation of Research Participants in High-Income Countries Who Lack Access to Health Care." *British Journal of Clinical Pharmacology* 81, no. 5 (2016): 857–64.

Dal-Ré, Rafael, Linda-Gail Bekker, Christian Gluud, and Nadarajah Sreeharan. "Ongoing and Future COVID-19 Vaccine Clinical Trials: Challenges and Opportunities." *The Lancet Infectious Diseases* 21, no. 6 (2021): 766–7.

Daniels, Norman. *Justice and Justification: Reflective Equilibrium in Theory and Practice*. New York: Cambridge University Press, 1996.

Daniels, Norman. "Accountability for Reasonableness." *British Medical Journal* 321, no. 7272 (2000): 1300–1.

Daniels, Norman. *Just Health: Meeting Health Needs Fairly*. Cambridge: Cambridge University Press, 2008.

Daniels, Norman. "A Progressively Realizable Right to Health and Global Governance." *Health Care Analysis* 23, no. 4 (2015): 330–40.

Daniels, Norman, and James E. Sabin. "Limits to Health Care: Fair Procedures, Democratic Deliberation, and the Legitimacy Problem for Insurers." *Philosophy and Public Affairs* 26, no. 4 (1997): 303–50.

Daniels, Norman, and James Sabin. *Setting Limits Fairly: Can We Learn to Share Medical Resources?* Oxford: Oxford University Press, 2002.

Daniels, Norman, John H. Bryant, Ramon A. Castaño, Octavio Gómez-Dantés, Kausar S. Khan, and Supasit Pannarunothai. "Benchmarks of Fairness for Health Care Reform: A Policy Tool for Developing Countries." *Bulletin of the World Health Organization* 78, no. 6 (2000): 740–50.

Del Savio, Lorenzo. "The Place of Crowdfunding in the Discovery of Scientific and Social Value of Medical Research." *Bioethics* 31, no. 5 (2017): 384–92.

Dickert, Neal, and Jeremy Sugarman. "Ethical Goals of Community Consultation in Research." *American Journal of Public Health* 95, no. 7 (2005): 1123–7.

Dresser, Rebecca. "Payments to Research Participants: the Importance of Context." *American Journal of Bioethics* 1, no. 2 (2001): 47.

Dupras, Charles, Marie-Pierre Dubé, Simon Gravel, and Hazar Haidar. "Accountability for Reasonableness as a Framework for the Promotion of Fair and Equitable Research." *Hastings Center Report* 54, no. S2 (2024): S66–S72.

Dworkin, Ronald. *Justice for Hedgehogs*. Cambridge, MA: Harvard University Press, 2011.

Elster, Jon. *Making Sense of Marx*. Cambridge: Cambridge University Press, 1985.

Elster, Jon. *Local Justice: How Institutions Allocate Scarce Goods and Necessary Burdens*. New York: Russell Sage Foundation, 1992.

Emanuel, Ezekiel J. "Benefits to Host Countries." In *The Oxford Textbook of Clinical Research Ethics*, edited by E. J. Emanuel et al., 719–28. Oxford: Oxford University Press, 2008.

Emanuel, Ezekiel J., and Participants in the 2001 Conference on Ethical Aspects of Research in Developing Countries. "Addressing Exploitation: Reasonable Availability Versus Fair Benefits." In *Exploitation and Developing Countries: The Ethics of Clinical Research*, edited by J. S. Hawkins and E. J. Emanuel, 286–313. Princeton, NJ: Princeton University Press, 2008.

Emanuel, Ezekiel J., Christine Grady, and David Wendler. "What Makes Clinical Research Ethical?" *JAMA* 283, no. 20 (2000): 2701–7.

Emanuel, Ezekiel J., David Wendler, Jack Killen, and Christine Grady. "What Makes Clinical Research in Developing Countries Ethical? The Benchmarks of Ethical Research." *The Journal of Infectious Diseases* 189, no. 5 (2004): 930–7.

European Federation of Pharmaceutical Industries and Associations. "The Pharmaceutical Industry in Figures 2024." 2024. https://www.efpia.eu/media/2rxdkn43/the-pharmaceutical-industry-in-figures-2024.pdf.

European Medicines Agency (EMA). "Twinrix Paediatirc." 2019. https://www.ema.europa.eu/en/medicines/human/EPAR/twinrix-paediatric#authorisation-detailssection [accessed April 4, 2026].

Expert Market Research. *Global Pharmaceuticals Market Analysis by Region and Key Companies*. Online report, 2023. https://www.expertmarketresearch.com/reports/pharmaceuticals-market.

Fagnan, Lyle J., Melinda Davis, Richard A. Deyo, James Werner, and Kurt Stange. "Linking Practice-Based Research Networks and Clinical and Translational Science Awards: New Opportunities for Community Engagement by Academic Health Centers." *Academic Medicine* 85, no. 3 (2010): 476–83.

Faunce, Thomas Alured, and Hitoshi Nasu. "Three Proposals for Rewarding Novel Health Technologies Benefiting People Living in Poverty: A Comparative Analysis of Prize Funds, Health Impact Funds and a Cost-Effectiveness/Competitive Tender Treaty." *Public Health Ethics* 1, no. 2 (2008): 146–53.

Feinberg, Joel. *The Moral Limits of The Criminal Law*. Volume 3: Harm to Self. New York: Oxford University Press, 1989.

Feinberg, Joel. *Harmless Wrongdoing*. Vol. 4. Oxford: Oxford University Press, 1990.

Ferguson, Benjamin et Zwolinski, Matt (eds.). *Exploitation: Perspectives from Philosophy, Politics, and Economics*. Oxford: Oxford University Press, 2024.

Fidler, David P. "Negotiating Equitable Access to Influenza Vaccines: Global Health Diplomacy and the Controversies Surrounding Avian Influenza H5N1 and Pandemic Influenza H1N1." *PLoS Medicine* 7, no. 5 (2010): e1000247.

Figueroa, J. Peter, Maria Elena Bottazzi, and Peter Hotez, Carolina Batista, Önder Ergonul, Sarah Gilbert, Mayda Gursel, Mazen Hassanain, Jerome H. Kim, Bhavna Lall, Heidi Larson, Denise Naniche, Timothy Sheahan, Shmuel Shoham, Annelies Wilder-Smith, Natalie Strub-Wourgaft, Prashant Yadav, and Gagandeep Kang. "Urgent Needs of Low-Income and Middle-Income Countries for COVID-19 Vaccines and Therapeutics." *The Lancet* 397, no. 10274 (2021): 562–4.

Finkel, Madelon L., Marleen Temmermann, Fatima Suleman, Michele Barry, Melissa Salm, Agnes Binagwaho and Peter H. Kilmarx. "What Do Global Health Practitioners Think About Decolonizing Global Health?" *Annals of Global Health* 88, no. 1 (2022): 61. https://pubmed.ncbi.nlm.nih.gov/33370211/.

Fisher, Jill A. *Medical Research for Hire: The Political Economy of Pharmaceutical Clinical Trials*. New Brunswick, NJ: Rutgers University Press, 2009.

Franco, Juan Víctor Ariel, and Karin Kopitowski. "Covid-19 Vaccine Trials in Low and Middle-Income Countries: What's the Benefit?". June 25, 2021. https://blogs.bmj.com/bmj/2021/06/25/covid-19-vaccine-trials-in-low-and-middle-income-countries-whats-the-benefit/.

Freedman, Benjamin. "Equipoise and the Ethics of Clinical Research." *The New England Journal of Medicine* 317, no. 3 (1987): 141–5.

Freeman, R. Edward. *Strategic Management: A Stakeholder Approach*. Cambridge University Press, 2010.

Freeman, Samuel R. *Rawls*. Abingdon: Taylor & Francis, 2007.

Fregonese, Federica. "Community Involvement in Biomedical Research Conducted in the Global Health Context; What Can Be Done to Make It Really Matter?" *BMC Medical Ethics* 19, no. Suppl 1 (2018): 44.

Friedman, Alex. "Beyond Accountability for Reasonableness." *Bioethics* 22, no. 2 (2008): 101–12.

Fries, James F., and Eswar Krishnan. "Equipoise, Design Bias, and Randomized Controlled Trials: The Elusive Ethics of New Drug Development." *Arthritis Research & Therapy* 6, no. 3 (2004): R250–R255.

Gauthier, David. *Morals by Agreement*. Oxford: Oxford University Press, 1986.

Gbadegesin, Segun et Wendler, David. "Protecting Communities in Health Research from Exploitation." *Bioethics* 20, no. 5 (2006): 248–53.

Gelling, Leslie. "Role of the Research Ethics Committee." *Nurse Education Today* 19, no. 7 (1999): 564–9.

George, Angella M., Rashid Ansumana, Dziedzom de Souza, Vettakkara K. Niyas, Alimuddin Zumla, and Moses J. Bockarie. "Climate Change and the Rising Incidence of Vector-Borne Diseases Globally." *International Journal of Infectious Diseases* 139 (2024): 143–5.

Geras, Norman. "Staying Home: G.A. Cohen and the Motivational Basis of Socialism." *Contemporary Politics* 19, no. 2 (2013): 234–46.

Gilabert, Pablo. "The Duty to Eradicate Global Poverty: Positive or Negative?" *Ethical Theory and Moral Practice* 7, no. 5 (2005): 537–50.

Gilbert, Margaret. "Obligation and Joint Commitment." *Utilitas* 11, no. 2 (1999): 143–63.

Gilbert, Margaret. *A Theory of Political Obligation: Membership, Commitment, and the Bonds of Society*. Oxford: Oxford University Press, 2006.

Gilead. "Full Efficacy and Safety Results for Gilead Investigational Twice-Yearly Lenacapavir for HIV Prevention Presented at AIDS 2024." 2024. https://www.gilead.com/news/news-details/2024/full-efficacy-and-safety-results-for-gilead-investigational-twice-yearly-lenacapavir-for-hiv-prevention-presented-at-aids-2024?utm_source=chatgpt.com.

Glantz, Leonard H., George J. Annas, Michael A. Grodin, and William K. Mariner. "Research in Developing Countries: Taking 'Benefit' Seriously." *The Hastings Center Report* 28, no. 6 (1998): 38–45.

Glickman, Seth W., John G. McHutchison, Eric D. Peterson, and Kevin A. Schulman. "Ethical and Scientific Implications of the Globalization of Clinical Research." *The New England Journal of Medicine* 360, no. 8 (2009): 816–23.

Global Forum on Bioethics in Research. "Dengue and Climate Change: Exploring Bioethical Challenges in Global Health Research." 2024, available at www.gfbr.global [accessed December 18, 2024].

Gold, Marthe R., Stevenson, David, et Fryback, Dennis G. "HALYS and QALYS and DALYS, Oh My: Similarities and Differences in Summary Measures of Population Health." *Annual Review of Public Health* 23, no. 1 (2002): 115–34.

Goodin, Robert. "Exploiting a Situation and Exploiting a Person." In *Modern Theories of Exploitation*, edited by A. Reeve, 166–200. London & Beverly Hills: Sage, 1987.

Grand View Research. "Pharmaceutical Market (2025–2030) Size, Share & Trends Analysis Report." 2025. https://www.grandviewresearch.com/industry-analysis/pharmaceutical-market-report.

Grant, Ruth W. et Sugarman, Jeremy. "Ethics in Human Subjects Research: Do Incentives Matter?" *The Journal of Medicine and Philosophy* 29, no. 6 (2004): 717–38.

Graves, Patricia M., and Myron M. Levine (eds.). *Battling Malaria: Strengthening the U.S. Military Malaria Vaccine Program*. Washington, DC: The National Academies Press, 2006.

Gray, Derrick. "Rethinking Micro-Level Exploitation." *Social Theory and Practice* (2020): 515–46.

Han Kun Newsletter. "Key Takeaways on 2022 China New Drug Clinical Trials Report." Han Kun Law Office. October 2023. https://www.hankunlaw.com/en/portal/article/index/cid/8/id/13674.html.

Hart, Herbert L. A. "Are There Any Natural Rights?" *The Philosophical Review* 64, no. 2 (1955): 175–91.

Hart, Herbert Lionel Adolphus et Honoré, Tony. *Causation in the Law*. Oxford: Oxford University Press, 1985.

Hart, Janelle. "Spotlight on China: A Dominant Player in the Clinical Trial Landscape." *Norstella*. 2024. https://www.norstella.com/spotlight-china/.

Hawkins, Jennifer S., and Ezekiel J. Emanuel. "Case Studies: The Havrix Trial and the Surfaxin Trial." In *Exploitation and Developing Countries: The Ethics of Clinical Research*, edited by J. S. Hawkins and E. J. Emanuel, 55–62. Princeton, NJ: Princeton University Press, 2008.

Heðinsdóttir, Katla. "Moving Beyond the Individualist Paradigm? Risse and Wollner on Non-agential Exploitation." *Moral Philosophy and Politics*, 9, no. 1 (2022): 51–67.

Heilinger, Jan-Christoph. *Cosmopolitan Responsibility: Global Injustice, Relational Equality, and Individual Agency*. Berlin: De Gruyter, 2019.

Held, David, and Pietro Maffettone. "Moral Cosmopolitanism and Democratic Values." Global Policy 8, no. S1 (2017): 54–64.

Hitchcock, Christopher. "Probabilistic Causation." *Stanford Encyclopaedia of Philosophy*. 2018, available at https://plato.stanford.edu/entries/causation-probabilistic/#ProbRaisTheoCaus [accessed April 8, 2026].

Hollis, Adrian. "Drugs for Neglected Diseases: New Incentives for Innovation." In *Pharmaceutical Innovation: Incentives, Competition, and Cost-Benefit Analysis in International Perspective*, edited by F. Sloan and C. Hsieh, 75–90. Cambridge: Cambridge University Press, 2007.

Hollis, Aidan. "The Health Impact Fund: A Useful Supplement to the Patent System?" *Public Health Ethics* 1, no. 2 (2008): 124–33.

Holzer, Felicitas. "International Patent Regimes and Access to Medicines: Is the Health Impact Fund an Effective Solution?" *Ordnung der Wissenschaft* 3, no. 1 (2016): 162–8.

Holzer, Felicitas. "Rawls and Social Value in Research." *The Hastings Center Report* 49, no. 2 (2019): 47.

Holzer, Felicitas S. "Defending the Social Value of Knowledge as a Safeguard for Public Trust." *Bioethics* 31, no. 7 (2017): 559–67.

Holzer, Felicitas, and Ignacio Mastroleo. "Ethical Aspects of Precision Medicine: an Introduction to the Ethics and Concept of Clinical Innovation." In *Precision Medicine: Tools and Quantitative Approaches*, edited by H. P. Deigner und M. Kohl, 1–19. Cambridge, MA: Academic Press, 2018.

Holzer, Felicitas, and Thomas Pogge. "The Health Impact Fund: Learning from COVID-19." In *COVID-19 in the Global South*, edited by Pádraig Carmody, Gerard McCann, Clodagh Colleran, and Ciara O'Halloran, 173–82. Bristol University Press, 2020.

Holzer, Felicitas, Tania Manríquez Roa, Federico Germani, Nikola Biller-Andorno, and Florencia Luna. "Charity or Empowerment? The Role of COVAX for Low and Middle-Income Countries." *Developing World Bioethics* 23, no. 1 (2023a): 59–66.

Holzer, Felicitas, Federico Germani, Ivette Ortiz, Nikola Biller-Andorno, and Julian März. "'VaxTax': A Follow-Up Proposal for a Global Vaccine Pandemic Response Fund." *Journal of Medical Ethics* 49, no. 3 (2023b): 160–4.

Homedes, Nuria, and Antonio Ugalde (eds.). *Clinical Trials in Latin America: Where Ethics and Business Clash*. New York: Springer, 2014.

Homedes, Núria, and Antonio Ugalde. "El ciclo de los medicamentos: su impacto en el acceso y el uso adecuado." *Salud colectiva* 11, no. 1 (2015): 5–8.

Homedes, Nuria, and Antonio Ugalde. "Ensayos Clínicos en América Latina: Implicancias para la Sustentabilidad y Seguridad de los Mercados Farmacéuticos y el Bienestar de los Sujetos." *Salud Colectiva* 12, no. 3 (2016): 317–45.

Hotez, Peter J., Serap Aksoy, and Paul J. Brindley. "Neglected Tropical Diseases: Progress Towards Addressing the Ancient Afflictions of Stigma and Poverty." *Trends in Parasitology* 38, no. 6 (2022): 439–45.

Hughes, Robert C. "Individual Risk and Community Benefit in International Research." *Journal of Medical Ethics* 38, no. 10 (2012): 626–9.

Hughes, Robert C. "Justifying Community Benefit Requirements in International Research." *Bioethics* 28, no. 8 (2014): 397–404.

Human Genome Organisation (HUGO) Ethics Committee. "Statement on Benefit-sharing." 2000. http://www.biobankresearch.org/governance-best-practice/statement-on-benefit-sharing/.

Hurst, Daniel J. "Benefit Sharing in a Global Context: Working Towards Solutions for Implementation." *Developing World Bioethics* 17, no. 2 (2017): 70–6.

Hurst, Samia. "Vulnerability in Old Age: The Fragility of Inappropriately Protected Interests." In *Aging and Human Nature: Perspectives from Philosophical, Theological, and Historical Anthropology*, edited by Mark Schweda, Michael Coors, and Claudia Bozzaro, 241–52. Cham: Springer Nature, 2020.

Hurst, Samia A. "Vulnerability in Research and Health Care; Describing the Elephant in the Room?" *Bioethics* 22, no. 4 (2008): 191–202.

Idämpään-Heikkilä, Juhana E., and Sev S. Fluss. "International Ethical Guidance from the Council for International Organizations of Medical Sciences." In *The Oxford Textbook of Clinical Research Ethics*, edited by E. J. Emanuel et al., 168–73. Oxford: Oxford University Press, 2008.

Igbokwe, Ezinne M., and Andrea Tosato. "Access to Medicines and Pharmaceutical Patents: Fulfilling the Promise of TRIPS Article 31bis." *Fordham Law Review* 91, no. 5 (2022): 1791–846.

Instituto Butantan. "A Parceria Tecnológica que Fez da CoronaVac a Vacina do Brasil." January 18, 2021. https://butantan.gov.br/noticias/a-parceria-tecnologica-que-fez-da-coronavac-a-vacina-do-brasil.

International Bioethics Committee (IBC). "Report of the IBC on the Principle of the Sharing of Benefits." 2015. https://unesdoc.unesco.org/ark:/48223/pf0000233230.

"Interview with Professor Natth." *Good Clinical Practice Journal* 6, no. 6 (1999): 11.

Jeske, Diane. "Special Obligations." *Stanford Encyclopedia of Philosophy*. 2021. https://plato.stanford.edu/entries/special-obligations/#2.

Jha, Prabhat, Anne Mills, Kara Hanson, Lilani Kumaranayake, Lesong Conteh, Christoph Kurowski, Son Nam Nguyen, Valeria Oliveira Cruz, Kent Ranson, Lara M. E. Vaz, Shengchao Yu, Oliver Morton, and Jeffrey D. Sachs. "Improving the Health of the Global Poor." *Science* 295, no. 5562 (2002): 2036–9.

John, Tyler M. et Millum, Joseph. "First Come, First Served?." *Ethics* 130, no. 2 (2020): 179–207.

Johnson, Robert, and Adam Cureton. "Kant's Moral Philosophy." *Stanford Encyclopedia of Philosophy*. 2016. https://plato.stanford.edu/entries/kant-moral/.

Jonas, Hans. "Philosophical Reflections on Experimenting with Human Subjects." *Daedalus: Journal of the American Academy of Arts and Sciences* 98, no. 2 (Spring 1969): 219–47

Kamuya, Dorcas M., Vicki Marsh, Patricia Njuguna, Patrick Munywoki, Michael Parker, and Sassy Molyneux. "'When They See Us, It's Like They Have Seen the Benefits!': Experiences of Study Benefits Negotiations in Community-Based Studies on the Kenyan Coast." *BMC Medical Ethics* 15, no. 1 (2014): 90.

Kant, Immanuel. *Groundwork for the Metaphysics of Morals*. Edited by J. B. Schneewind. New Haven, CT: Yale University Press, 2002.

Kapiriri, Lydia, James V. Lavery, Peter A. Singer, Hassan Mshinda, Lorne Babiuk, and Abdallah S. Daar. "The Case for Conducting First-in-Human (Phase 0 and Phase 1) Clinical Trials in Low and Middle Income Countries." *BMC Public Health* 11, no. 1 (2011): 811.

Kho, Michelle E., Ellen Rawski, Julie Makarski, and Melissa C. Brouwers. "Recruitment of Multiple Stakeholders to Health Services Research: Lessons from the Front Lines." *BMC Health Services Research* 10, no. 1 (2010): 123.

Kime, Megan. "Theories of Global Justice: Relational and Non-Relational Approaches." PhD thesis, University of Leeds, 2009. http://etheses.whiterose.ac.uk/14531/1/521864.pdf.

Kimmelman, Jonathan, and Alex John London. "The Structure of Clinical Translation: Efficiency, Information, and Ethics." *The Hastings Center Report* 45, no. 2 (2015): 27–39.

King, Katherine F., Pamela Kolopack, Maria W. Merritt, and James Lavery. "Community Engagement and the Human Infrastructure of Global Health Research." *BMC Medical Ethics* 15, no. 1 (2014): 84.

Kitcher, Philip. *Science in a Democratic Society*. Buffalo, NY: Prometheus Books, 2011.

Kleingeld, Pauline, and Eric Brown. "Cosmopolitanism." *Stanford Encyclopaedia of Philosophy*. 2013, available at https://plato.stanford.edu/entries/cosmopolitanism/ [accessed March 18, 2026].

Kleingeld, Pauline, and Eric Brown. "Cosmopolitanism." In *The Stanford Encyclopedia of Philosophy* (Winter 2024 Edition), edited by Edward N. Zalta and Uri Nodelman. https://plato.stanford.edu/archives/win2024/entries/cosmopolitanism/.

Klosko, George. "Political Obligation and Gratitude." *Philosophy & Public Affairs* 18, no. 4 (1989): 352–8.

Klosko, George. *The Principle of Fairness and Political Obligation*. 2nd ed. Lanham, MD: Rowman & Littlefield, 1992.

Klosko, George. *Political Obligations*. Oxford: Oxford University Press, 2005.

Klosko, George. "Fairness Obligations and Non-Acceptance of Benefits." *Political Studies* 62, no. 1 (2014): 159–71.

Kohli, Amit. "Novartis, Die Obdachlosen und Die Vogelgrippe." *Public Eye Magazine*. April 2016.

Kolata, Gina, and Kurt Eichenwald. "Stopgap Medicine: A Special Report. For the Uninsured, Drug Trials Are Health Care." *The New York Times*. June 22 1999, available at http://www.nytimes.com/1999/06/22/business/stopgap-medicine-a-special-report-for-the-uninsureddrug-trials-are-health-care.html [accessed March 7, 2026].

Kukla, Rebecca. "Resituating the Principle of Equipoise: Justice and Access to Care in Non-Ideal Conditions." *Kennedy Institute of Ethics Journal* 17, no. 3 (2007): 171–202.

Kutz, Christopher. *Complicity: Ethics and Law for a Collective Age*. Cambridge: Cambridge University Press, 2000.

Kwete, Xiaoxiao, Kun Tang, Lucy Chen, Ran Ren, Qi Chen, Zhenru Wu, Yi Cai, and Hao Li. "Decolonizing Global Health: What Should Be the Target of This Movement and Where Does It Lead Us?" *Global Health Research and Policy* 7, no. 1 (2022): 3.

Lairumbi, Geoffrey M., Michael Parker, Raymond Fitzpatrick, and Michael English. "Forms of Benefit Sharing in Global Health Research Undertaken in Resource Poor Settings: A Qualitative Study of Stakeholders' Views in Kenya." *Philosophy, Ethics, and Humanities in Medicine* 7, no. 1 (2012): 7.

Lamont, Julian. "Distributive Justice." *Stanford Encyclopedia of Philosophy*. 2017a. https://plato.stanford.edu/entries/justice-distributive/.

Lamont, Julian. *Distributive Justice*. London: Routledge, 2017b.

Langlois, Adele. "The UNESCO Universal Declaration on Bioethics and Human Rights: Perspectives from Kenya and South Africa." *Health Care Analysis* 16, no. 1 (2008): 39–51.

Laurion, Victor et Robertson, Christopher. "Why the Duty to Research Falls on Institutions Rather than Individuals." *The American Journal of Bioethics* 19, no. 6 (2019): 44–6.

Lavery, James V., Sunita VS Bandewar, Joshua Kimani, Ross Upshur, Frances Plummer, and Peter Singer. "'Relief of Oppression': An Organizing Principle for Researchers' Obligations to Participants in Observational Studies in the Developing World." *BMC Public Health* 10, no. 1 (2010): 384.

Lawrence, Carlton et Stewart, Kearsley. "The Challenge of Community Representation: Lessons from Six HIV Clinical Research Community Advisory Boards in Uganda." *Journal of Empirical Research on Human Research Ethics* 11, no. 4 (2016): 311–21.

Ledford, Heidi. "Edits to Ethics Code Rankle." *Nature* 515, no. 7526 (2014): 174.

Lee, Eric. "Our Flawed Approach to Undue Inducement in Medical Research." *Bioethics* 33, no. 4 (2019): 13–18.

Lee, Vivian Chia-Jou, Jacqueline Yao, and William Zhang. "The Health Impact Fund: Making the Case for Engagement with Pharmaceutical Laboratories in Brazil, Russia, India, and China." *Globalization and Health* 17, no. 1 (2021): 101.

Lester, Jan C. "*Against Against Intellectual Property*: A Short Refutation of Meme Communism." 2016. https://philarchive.org/archive/LESAAI [accessed March 18, 2026].

Levine, Robert J. "The Nature, Scope, and Justification of Clinical Research." In *The Oxford Textbook of Clinical Research Ethics*, edited by E. J. Emanuel et al., 211–21. Oxford: Oxford University Press, 2008.

Li, Zhanpeng, and Peng Guo. "Compulsory Licensing of Pharmaceuticals During Public Health Crisis: A TRIPS Framework Analysis." *Frontiers in Public Health* 13 (2025): 1630586.

Lie, Reidar K. *Justice and International Research. Biomedical Research Ethics: Updating International Guidelines*. Geneva: A consultation, 2000: 27–39.

Livemint. "How Many Countries Have Recognised Covishield, Covaxin? Health Minister Answers." November 20, 2021. https://www.livemint.com/news/india/how-many-countries-have-recognised-covishield-covaxin-health-minister-answers-11636508481586.html?utm_source=chatgpt.com.

London, Alex J. "Justice and the Human Development Approach to International Research." *The Hastings Center Report* 35, no. 1 (2005): 24–37.

London, Alex J. "Responsiveness to Host Community Health Needs." In *The Oxford Textbook of Clinical Research Ethics*, edited by E. J. Emanuel et al., 737–46. Oxford: Oxford University Press, 2008.

London, Alex J. "Non-Paternalistic Model of Research Ethics and Oversight: Assessing the Benefits of Prospective Review." *Journal of Law Medicine & Ethics* 40, no. 202 (2012): 930–44.

London, Alex John, and Jonathan Kimmelman. "Justice in Translation: From Bench to Bedside in the Developing World." *The Lancet* 372, no. 9632 (2008): 82–5.

London, Alex John et Zollman, Kevin J. S. "Research at the Auction Block: Problems for the Fair Benefits Approach to International Research." *Hastings Center Report* 40, no. 4 (2010): 34–45.

London, Alex John, Kimmelman, Jonathan, et Emborg, Marina Elena. "Beyond Access vs. Protection in Trials of Innovative Therapies." *Science* 328, no. 5980 (2010): 829–30.

Luna, Florencia. "Elucidating the Concept of Vulnerability: Layers Not Labels." *IJFAB: International Journal of Feminist Approaches to Bioethics* 2, no. 1 (2009): 121–39.

Luna, Florencia. "Identifying and Evaluating Layers of Vulnerability – a Way Forward." *Developing World Bioethics* 19, no. 2 (2019): 86–95.

Luna, Florencia, and Felicitas Holzer. "What Vaccine Inequity Has Taught Us: A Way Forward Through the Lens of Ideal and Non-Ideal Theory." *Global Bioethics* 36, no. 1 (2025): 2497602.

Lurie, Peter, and Sidney M. Wolfe. "Unethical Trials of Interventions to Reduce Perinatal Transmission of the Human Immunodeficiency Virus in Developing Countries." *The New England Journal of Medicine* 337, no. 12 (1997): 853–6.

Macdonald, Chris et Walton, Nancy. "The Perverse Consequences of a Proposed Global Tax on Research." *The American Journal of Bioethics* 10, no. 6 (2010): 46–7.

Macklin, Ruth. "Due and Undue Inducements: On Paying Money to Research Subjects." *IRB: Ethics & Human Research* 3, no. 5 (1981): 1–6.

Macklin, Ruth. *Double Standards in Medical Research in Developing Countries*. Vol. 2. Cambridge: Cambridge University Press, 2004a.

Macklin, Ruth. "Ética de la Investigación Internacional: el Problema de la Justicia hacia los Países menos Desarrollados." *Acta Bioethica* 10, no. 1 (2004b): 27–36.

Macklin, Ruth. "Standard of Care: An Evolution in Ethical Thinking." *The Lancet* 372, no. 9635 (2008): 284–5.

Macklin, Ruth. "Fair Benefits in Developing Countries: Maximin as a Good Start." *The American Journal of Bioethics* 10, no. 6 (2010): 36–7.

Macklin, Ruth. "The 'Responsiveness Requirement' Defended in Post-Trial Access to Trial Drugs: Legal, Ethical, and Practical Issues." Workshop, 2011. http://ptaworkshop.files.wordpress.com/2012/01/responsiveness_requirement_defended.pdf.

Macqueen, Kathleen M., Anant Bhan, Janet Frohlich, J. Holzer, and Jeremy Sugarman. "Evaluating Community Engagement in Global Health Research: The Need for Metrics." *BMC Medical Ethics* 16, no. 1 (2015): 44.

Malmqvist, Erik. "Taking Advantage of Injustice." *Social Theory and Practice* 39, no. 4 (2013): 557–80.

Malmqvist, Erik. "Better to Exploit than to Neglect? International Clinical Research and the Non-Worseness Claim." *Journal of Applied Philosophy* 34, no. 4 (2017): 474–88.

Malmqvist, Erik, and András Szigeti. "Exploitation and Joint Action." *Journal of Social Philosophy* 50, no. 3 (2019): 280–300.

Malmqvist, Erik, and András Szigeti. "Exploitation and Remedial Duties." *Journal of Applied Philosophy* 38, no. 1 (2021): 55–72.

Manne, Kate. *Down Girl: The Logic of Misogyny*. Oxford: Oxford University Press, 2017.

MARCAD Consortium. "About MARCAD." n.d. Retrieved December 8, 2025, from https://www.marcad-africa.org/.

Markovits, Daniel. "Market Solidarity: Price as Commensuration, Contract as Integration." *Working paper*, 2017, online available at iast.fr/sites/default/files/IAST/conf/law/markovits2018bis.pdf [accessed August 17, 2025].

Marmot, Michael G. et Wilkinson, Richard G. (eds.). *Social Determinants of Health: The Solid Facts*. Copenhagen: World Health Organization, 2003.

Marshall, Elliot. "Lemons, Oranges, and Complexity." *Science* 322, no. 5899 (2008): 209.

Martin, Angela et Hurst, Samia. "On Vulnerability—Analysis and Applications of a Many-faceted Concept: Introduction." *Les ateliers de l'éthique* 12, no. 2 (2017): 146–53.

Mayer, Robert. "Sweatshops, Exploitation, and Moral Responsibility." *Journal of Social Philosophy* 38, no. 4 (2007): 605–19.

McKeown, Maeve. "Global Structural Exploitation: Towards an Intersectional Definition." *Global Justice: Theory Practice Rhetoric* 9, no. 2 (2016): 155–77.

McMillan, John. "Human Rights: The Normative Engine of Fairness and Research in Developing Countries." *The American Journal of Bioethics* 10, no. 6 (2010): 47–9.

Meckled-Garcia, Saladin. "The Practice-Dependence Red Herring and Better Reasons for Restricting the Scope of Justice." *Raisons Politiques* 1, no. 3 (2013): 97–120.

Meketa, Irina. "Honor Among (the Beneficiaries of) Thieves." *Ethical Theory and Moral Practice* 18, no. 2 (2014): 385–402.

Merritt, Maria W. "Health Researchers' Ancillary Care Obligations in Low-Resource Settings: How Can We Tell What Is Morally Required?" *Kennedy Institute of Ethics Journal* 21, no. 4 (2011): 311–47.

Merritt, Maria W., Taylor, Holly A., et Mullany, Luke C. "Ancillary Care in Community-based Public Health Intervention Research." *American Journal of Public Health* 100, no. 2 (2010): 211–16.

Miller, David. *Social Justice*. Oxford: Clarendon Press, 1976.

Miller, David. *Market, State, and Community*. Oxford: Clarendon Press, 1989.

Miller, David. "Distributing Responsibilities." *The Journal of Political Philosophy* 9, no. 4 (2001a): 453–71.

Miller, David. *Principles of Social Justice*. Cambridge MA: Harvard University Press, 2001b.

Miller, David. "National Responsibility and Global Justice." *Critical Review of International Social and Political Philosophy* 11, no. 4 (2008): 383–99. DOI: 10.1080/13698230802415862.

Millum, Joseph. "Post-Trial Access to Antiretrovirals: Who Owes What to Whom?" *Bioethics* 25, no. 3 (2011): 145–54.

Millum, Joseph. "Sharing the Benefits of Research Fairly: Two Approaches." *Journal of Medical Ethics* 38, no. 4 (2012): 219–23.
Millum, Joseph, Megan Campbell, Florencia Luna, Arianne Malekzadeh, and Q. Abdool Karim. "Ethical Challenges in Global Health-Related Stigma Research." *BMC Medicine* 17, no. 1 (2019): 84.
Milne, Heather. "Desert, Effort and Equality." *Journal of Applied Philosophy* 3, no. 2 (1986): 235–43.
Mitra, Agomoni Ganguli. "Off-Shoring Clinical Research: Exploitation and the Reciprocity Constraint." *Developing World Bioethics* 13, no. 3 (2012): 111–18.
Montero, Julio. *Human Rights as Human Independence: A Philosophical and Legal Interpretation*. Philadelphia: University of Pennsylvania Press, 2022.
Multi Regional Clinical Trials (MRCT) Center. "Post-Trial Responsibilities Framework: Continued Access to Investigational Medicines Guidance Document." 2017, available at https://mrctcenter.org/wp-content/uploads/2017/12/2017-12-07-Post-Trial-Responsibilities-Guidance-Document-Version-1.2.pdf [accessed March 18, 2026].
Mulumba, Moses, Jessica Oga, Nana Koomson, Tasha-Aliya Kara, Adanze Nge Cynthia, and Lisa Forman. "Decolonizing Global Health: Africa's Pursuit of Pharmaceutical Sovereignty." *BMC Health Services Research* 25, no. 1 (2025): 1015.
Murphy, Jill, Jennifer Hatfield, Kaosar Afsana, and Vic Neufeld. "Making a Commitment to Ethics in Global Health Research Partnerships: A Practical Tool to Support Ethical Practice." *Journal of Bioethical Inquiry* 12, no. 1 (2015): 137–46.
Murray, Pete. "Allocative Justice." In *The Cambridge Rawls Lexicon*, edited by J. Mandle and D. A. Reidy, 7–8. Cambridge: Cambridge University Press, 2015.
National Bioethics Advisory Commission (NBAC). "Ethical and Policy Issues in International Research Involving Human Participants." 2001a, available at https://bioethicsarchive.georgetown.edu/nbac/human/overvol1.pdf [accessed March 18, 2026].
National Bioethics Advisory Commission (NBAC). "When Research Is Concluded – Access to the Benefits of Research by Participants, Communities, and Countries." *Ethical and Policy Issues in International Research: Clinical Trials in Developing Countries*. 2001b, available at https://bioethicsarchive.georgetown.edu/nbac/clinical/Chapter4.pdf [accessed March 18, 2026].
National Commission for the Protection of Human Subjects of Biomedical and Behavioral Research. "The Belmont Report: Ethical Principles and Guidelines for the Protection of Human Subjects of Research." 1979. https://www.hhs.

gov/ohrp/regulations-and-policy/belmont-report/read-the-belmont-report/index.html.

New Drug Approvals. "BBIBP CorV, Sinopharm COVID 19 Vaccine." March 23, 2021. https://newdrugapprovals.org/2021/03/23/bbibp-corv-sinopharm-covid-19-vaccine/.

Normile, Dennis. "The Promise and Pitfalls of Clinical Trials Overseas." *Science* 322, no. 5899 (2008): 214–16.

Nozick, Robert. *Anarchy, State, and Utopia*. Malden, MA: Basic Books, 1974.

Nussbaum, Marta C. "Nature, Function, and Capability: Aristotle on Political Distribution." In *Aristoteles' 'Politik'*, edited by G. Patzig, 152–86. Gottingen: Vandenhoeck and Ruprecht, 1990.

Nussbaum, Marta C. "Non-Relative Virtues: An Aristotelian Approach." In *The Quality of Life*, edited by M. C. Nussbaum and A. Sen, 242–79. Oxford: Clarendon Press, 1993.

Nussbaum, Marta C. "Patriotism and Cosmopolitanism." *Boston Review* 19, no. 5 (1994), 1–8, online available at chrome-extension://efaidnbmnnnibpcajpcglclefindmkaj/https://bordeure.wordpress.com/wp-content/uploads/2008/09/patriotism-and-cosmopolitanism.pdf [accessed March 18, 2026].

Nussbaum, Marta C. "Capabilities and Human Rights." *Fordham Law Review* 66, no. 2 (1997): 273–300.

Nussbaum, Marta C., and Amartya Sen (eds.). *The Quality of Life*. Oxford: Clarendon Press, 1993.

O'Neill, Onora. *Towards Justice and Virtue: A Constructive Account of Practical Reasoning*. Cambridge: Cambridge University Press, 1996.

Okonta, Patrick I. "Ethics of Clinical Trials in Nigeria." *Nigerian Medical Journal* 55, no. 3 (2014): 188–94.

Ooms, Gorik, David Stuckler, Sanjay Basu, and Martin McKee. "Financing the Millennium Development Goals for Health and Beyond: Sustaining the 'Big Push.'" *Globalization and Health* 6, no. 1 (2010): 17.

Oxford Dictionary. "Community." 2024. https://en.oxforddictionaries.com/definition/community.

Pallikkathayil, Japa. "Cosmopolitanism and the Evolution of Institutions." *Philosophy* (2025): 1–17.

Parfit, Derek. *On What Matters*. Vol. 1. Oxford: Oxford University Press, 2011.

Participants in the 2001 Conference on Ethical Aspects of Research in Developing Countries. "Moral Standards for Research in Developing Countries: From 'Reasonable Availability' to 'Fair Benefits.'" *The Hastings Center Report* 34, no. 3 (2004): 17–27.

Patten, Alan. "Should We Stop Thinking About Poverty in Terms of Helping the Poor?" *Ethics & International Affairs* 19, no. 1 (2005): 19–27.

Paul Ehrlich Institute. "Hepatitis-A-Impfstoffe." 2019, available at https://www.pei.de/DE/arzneimittel/impfstoff-impfstoffe-fuer-den-menschen/hepatitis-a/hepatitis-aalle-table.html [accessed April 4, 2026].

Pearl, Judea. *Causality: Models, Reasoning, and Inference*. Cambridge: Cambridge University Press, 2000.

Petryna, Adriana. *When Experiments Travel: Clinical Trials and the Global Search for Human Subjects*. Princeton, NJ: Princeton University Press, 2009.

Phillips, Robert A. "Stakeholder Theory and a Principle of Fairness." *Business Ethics Quarterly* 7, no. 1 (1997): 51–66.

Pogge, Thomas. *World Poverty and Human Rights*. Cambridge: Polity Press, 2002.

Pogge, Thomas. "Human Rights and Global Health: A Research Program." *Metaphilosophy* 36, no. 1–2 (2005a): 182–209.

Pogge, Thomas. "World Poverty and Human Rights." *Ethics & International Affairs* 19, no. 1 (2005b): 1–7.

Pogge, Thomas. "Access to Medicines." *Public Health Ethics* 1, no. 2 (2008): 73–82.

Pogge, Thomas. "The Health Impact Fund and Its Justification by Appeal to Human Rights." *Journal of Social Philosophy* 40, no. 4 (2009): 542–69.

Pogge, Thomas et Laukötter, Sebastian. "Menschenrechte, Weltgesundheit und unsere Verantwortung: Thomas Pogge (Yale) im Gespräch mit Sebastian Laukötter (Münster)." *Ethik in der Medizin* 25, no. 2 (2013): 157–63.

Porter, Joan P., and Greg Koski. "Regulations for the Protection of Humans in Research in the United States." In *The Oxford Textbook of Clinical Research Ethics*, edited by E. J. Emanuel et al., 156–73. Oxford: Oxford University Press, 2008.

Post, Stephen G. (ed.) *Encyclopedia of Bioethics*. Chicago, IL: MacMillan, 2003.

Pratt, Bridget. "Research for Health Justice: An Ethical Framework Linking Global Health Research to Health Equity." *BMJ Global Health* 6, no. 2 (2021): 1–15.

Pratt, Bridget, and Bebe Loff. "Framework to Link International Clinical Research to the Promotion of Justice in Global Health." *Bioethics* 28, no. 8 (2013): 387–96.

Pratt, Bridget et Loff, Bebe. "A Framework to Link International Clinical Research to the Promotion of Justice in Global Health." *Bioethics* 28, no. 8 (2014): 387–96.

Pratt, Bridget, and Adnan A. Hyder. "Reinterpreting Responsiveness for Health Systems Research in Low and Middle Income Countries." *Bioethics* 29, no. 6 (2015): 379–88.

Pratt, Bridget et Hyder, Adnan A. "Fair Resource Allocation to Health Research: Priority Topics for Bioethics Scholarship." *Bioethics* 31, no. 6 (2017): 454–66.

Pratt, Bridget et De Vries, Jantina. "Community Engagement in Global Health Research That Advances Health Equity." *Bioethics* 32, no. 7 (2018): 454–63.

Pratt, Bridget, Mark Sheehan, Nicola Barsdorf, and Adnan A. Hyder. "Exploring the Ethics of Global Health Research Priority-Setting." *BMC Medical Ethics* 19, no. 1 (2018): 94.

Ratto-Kim, Silvia, In-Kyu Yoon, Robert M. Paris, Jean-Louis Excler, Jerome H. Kim, and Robert J. O'Connell "The US Military Commitment to Vaccine Development: A Century of Successes and Challenges." *Frontiers in Immunology* 9 (2018): 1397.

Ravvin, Michael. "Incentivizing Access and Innovation for Essential Medicines: A Survey of the Problem and Proposed Solutions." *Public Health Ethics* 1, no. 2 (2008): 110–23.

Rawls, John. "Justice as Fairness." *The Philosophical Review* 67, no. 2 (1958): 164–94.

Rawls, John. "Legal Obligation and the Duty of Fair Play." In *Law and Philosophy*, edited by S. Hook, 117–29. New York: New York University Press, 1964.

Rawls, John. *A Theory of Justice* [TJ]. Cambridge, MA: Harvard University Press, 1971.

Rawls, John. *A Theory of Justice*. Revised ed. [TJR]. Cambridge, MA: Harvard University Press, 1999a.

Rawls, John. *The Law of Peoples* [LP]. Cambridge, MA: Harvard University Press, 1999b.

Rawls, John. *Justice as Fairness: A Restatement* [JF]. Edited by Erin Kelly. Cambridge, MA: Harvard University Press, 2001.

Reeve, Andrew. *Modern Theories of Exploitation*. London & Beverly Hills: Sage, 1987.

Rehfeld, Andrew. "Book Review on Klosko, George: The Principle of Fairness and Political Obligation." *Ethics* 104, no. 2 (2005): 418–22.

Reichenbach, Hans. *The Direction of Time*. Berkeley and Los Angeles: University of California Press, 1956.

Resnik, David B. "The Ethics of HIV Research in Developing Nations." *Bioethics* 12, no. 4 (1998): 286–306.

Resnik, David B. "Exploitation in Biomedical Research." *Theoretical Medicine and Bioethics* 24, no. 3 (2003): 233–59.

Resnik, David B. "Practical and Political Problems with a Global Research Tax." *The American Journal of Bioethics* 10, no. 6 (2010): 44–5.

Resnik, David B. "Examining the Social Benefits Principle in Research with Human Participants." *Health Care Analysis* 26, no. 1 (2016): 66–80.

Resnik, Michael D. *Choices: An Introduction to Decision Theory*. Minneapolis: University of Minnesota Press, 1987.

Richardson, Henry S. *Moral Entanglements: The Ancillary-Care Obligations of Medical Researchers*. Oxford: Oxford University Press, 2012.

Riley, Jonathan. "Justice Under Capitalism." In *Markets and Justice*, edited by J. W. Chapman, 122–62. New York: New York University Press, 1989.

Risse, Mathias. "Do We Owe the Global Poor Assistance or Rectification?" *Ethics and International Affairs* 19, no. 1 (2005): 9–18.

Rivera Lopez, Eduardo. "Explotación y Bioética. Ética Individual y Regulación Jurídica." *Revista de Bioética y Derecho* 40 (2017): 7–22.

Rocklöv, Joacim, and Yesim Tozan. "Climate Change and the Rising Infectiousness of Dengue." *Emerging Topics in Life Sciences* 3, no. 2 (2019): 133–42.

Roemer, John E. *Egalitarian Perspectives: Essays in Philosophical Economics*. Cambridge: Cambridge University Press, 1996.

Ruger, Jennifer Prah. "Health and Social Justice." *The Lancet* 364, no. 9439 (2004): 1075–80.

Ruger, Jennifer Prah. *Health and Social Justice*. Oxford: Oxford University Press, 2008.

Ruger, Jennifer Prah. "Global Health Justice." *Public Health Ethics* 2, no. 3 (2009): 261–75.

Sadurski, Wojciech. *Giving Desert Its Due: Social Justice and Legal Theory*. Dordrecht: D. Reidel, 1985.

Sample, Ruth J. *Exploitation: What It Is and Why It's Wrong*. Lanham, MD: Rowman & Littlefield, 2003.

Sample, Ruth. "Structural Exploitation and Expressive Content." In *Presentation at the Workshop "Exploitation in Bioethics"* (2018). University of Copenhagen, November 2018.

Sangiovanni, Andrea. "Global Justice, Reciprocity, and the State." *Philosophy & Public Affairs* 35, no. 1 (2007): 3–39.

Savulescu, Julian. "The Fiction of 'Undue Inducement': Why Researchers Should Be Allowed to Pay Participants Any Amount of Money for Any Reasonable Research Project." *American Journal of Bioethics* 1, no. 2 (2001): 1–3.

Schroeder, Doris. "Benefit Sharing: It's Time for a Definition." *Journal of Medical Ethics* 33, no. 4 (2007): 205–9.

Schroeder, Doris. "Sharing of Benefits." In *Handbook of Global Bioethics*, edited by Henk ten Have and Bert Gordijn, 203–23. New York: Springer, 2014.

Schroeder, Doris, Julie Cook Lucas, Francois Hirsch, Solveig Fenet, and Vasantha Muthuswamy. *Ethics Dumping: Case Studies from North-South Research Collaborations*. Cham: Springer, 2018.

Schuklenk, Udo. "For-Profit Clinical Trials in Developing Countries—Those Troublesome Patient Benefits." *The American Journal of Bioethics* 10, no. 6 (2010): 52–4.

Schulz-Baldes, Annette, Vayena, Effy, et Biller-Andorno, Nikola. "Sharing Benefits in International Health Research." *Research-Capacity Building as an Example of an Indirect Collective Benefit*. EMBO reports, 8, no. 1 (2007): 8.

Schütz, Elna. "'Miraculous' HIV Drug to Be Rolled Out After Overcoming Aid Cuts Threat." *BMJ* 391 (2025). https://doi.org/10.1136/bmj.r2452.

Sen, Amartya. *Poverty and Famines*. Oxford: Clarendon Press, 1981.

Sen, Amartya. "Capability and Well-Being." In *The Quality of Life*, edited by Marta C. Nussbaum and Armartya Sen, 30–53. Oxford: Clarendon Press, 1993.

Sen, Amartya. *Development as Freedom*. New York: Knopf, 1999.

Sethuraman, K. Raman. "Scientific Imperialism and 'Safari Research.'" *BMJ* (2001), online available at https://www.bmj.com/rapid-response/2011/10/28/scientific-imperialism-and-safari-research [accessed March 13, 2026].

Shinde, Viraj A., Ramanand Patil, Prasan Bhandari, Prachitee Borkar, and Shraddha Yadav. "A Pharmacoeconomic Outlook of the Biological Drugs Marketed in India: A Cost Variance Analysis." *Cureus* 15, no. 1 (2023): e33943.

Shue, Henry. *Basic Rights: Subsistence, Affluence, and US Foreign Policy*. Princeton, NJ: Princeton University Press, 1996.

Sidgwick, Henry. *The Methods of Ethics*. 7th ed. London: Macmillan, 1907.

Silver, Andrew. "China Approves CSPC Pharma mRNA Cancer Therapy for Clinical Trials." Reuters. June 25, 2024. https://www.reuters.com/business/healthcare-pharmaceuticals/china-approves-cspc-pharma-mrna-cancer-therapy-clinical-trials-2024-06-26/.

Simmons, A. John. "The Principle of Fair Play." *Philosophy & Public Affairs* 8, no. 4 (1979a): 307–37.

Simmons, A. John. *Moral Principles and Political Obligations*. Princeton, NJ: Princeton University Press, 1979b.

Simmons, A. John. *Justification and Legitimacy: Essays on Rights and Obligations*. Cambridge: Cambridge University Press, 2001.

Singal, Amit G., Peter D. Higgins, and Akbar K. Waljee. "A Primer on Effectiveness and Efficacy Trials." *Clinical and Translational Gastroenterology* 5, no. 1 (2014): e45.

Singer, Peter. "Famine, Affluence, and Morality." *Philosophy and Public Affairs* 1, no. 3 (1972): 229–43.

Singer, Peter. *The Life You Can Save: How to Do Your Part to End World Poverty*. New York: Random House Trade Paperbacks, 2009.

Sinovac Biotech Ltd. "South Africa Phase III Clinical Study Shows SINOVAC CoronaVac® Safe for Children as Young as 6 Months." Press release. December 29, 2021. https://www.sinovac.com/en-us/news/id-3036.

Snyder, Jeremy. "Exploitations and Their Complications: The Necessity of Identifying the Multiple Forms of Exploitation in Pharmaceutical Trials." *Bioethics* 26, no. 5 (2012): 251–8.

Sonderholm, Jorn. "A Reform Proposal in Need of Reform: A Critique of Thomas Pogge's Proposal for How to Incentivize Research and Development of Essential Drugs." *Public Health Ethics* 3, no. 2 (2010): 167–77.

Sonderholm, Jorn. "Thomas Pogge on Global Justice and World Poverty: A Review Essay." *Analytic Philosophy* 53, no. 4 (2012): 366–91.

Spector, Céline. "Rawls et le Devoir de Fair Play." *Philosophical Enquiries: Revue des Philosophies Anglophones*. 2014, available at https://hal.sorbonne-universite.fr/hal-01940429/document [accessed September 19, 2025].

Stilz, Anna. "Collective Responsibility and the State." *Journal of Political Philosophy* 19, no. 2 (2011): 190–208.

Suppes, Patrick. *A Probabilistic Theory of Causality*. Amsterdam: North-Holland Publishing, 1970.

Tagoe, Nadia, Sassy Molyneux, Justin Pulford, and Sam Kinyanjui. "Consortium Management Structures, Processes, and Approaches: The DELTAS Africa Example." *Wellcome Open Research* 7 (2023): 139.

Temkin, Larry S. "Thinking About the Needy, Justice, and International Organizations." *The Journal of Ethics* 8, no. 4 (2004): 349–95.

The Nuremberg Code. "The Nuremberg Code. Trials of War Criminals Before the Nuremberg Military Tribunals Under Control Council Law." 1949. https://history.nih.gov/research/downloads/nuremberg.pdf.

'T Hoen, Ellen F. M., Tapiwanashe Kujinga, and Pascale Boulet. "Patent Challenges in the Procurement and Supply of Generic New Essential Medicines and Lessons from HIV in the Southern African Development Community (SADC) Region." *Journal of Pharmaceutical Policy and Practice* 11 (2018): 31.

Tosi, Justin. "Rethinking the Principle of Fair Play." *Pacific Philosophical Quarterly* 99, no. 4 (2018): 612–31.

Tully, Danielle, and Carrie L. Griffiths. "Dengvaxia: The World's First Vaccine for Prevention of Secondary Dengue." *Therapeutic Advances in Vaccines and Immunotherapy* 9 (2021): 1–8.

United Nations Educational, Scientific, and Cultural Organization (UNESCO). "Universal Declaration on Bioethics and Human Rights." 2005. http://portal.unesco.org/en/ev.php-URL_ID=31058&URL_DO=DO_TOPIC&URL_SECTION=201.html.

United Nations Educational, Scientific, and Cultural Organization (UNESCO). "International Bioethics Committee (IBC)." 2019. http://www.unesco.org/new/en/social-and-human-sciences/themes/bioethics/international-bioethics-committee/.

Valdman, Mikhail. "Exploitation and Injustice." *Social Theory and Practice* 34, no. 4 (2008): 551–72.

Valdman, Mikhail. "A Theory of Wrongful Exploitation." *Philosophers' Imprint* 9, no. 6 (2009): 1–14.

Van Buren, Harry J. "If Fairness Is the Problem, Is Consent the Solution? Integrating ISCT and Stakeholder Theory." *Business Ethics Quarterly* 11, no. 3 (2001): 481–99.

Varmus, Harold, and David Satcher. "Ethical Complexities of Conducting Research in Developing Countries." *The New England Journal of Medicine* 337, no. 14 (1997): 1003–5.

Venkatapuram, Sridhar et Marmot, Michael. "Epidemiology and Social Justice in Light of Social Determinants of Health Research." *Bioethics* 23, no. 2 (2009): 79–89.

Vrousalis, Nicholas. "Exploitation, Vulnerability, and Social Domination." *Philosophy & Public Affairs* 41, no. 2 (2013): 131–57.

Vrousalis, Nicholas. "G.A. Cohen on Exploitation." *Politics, Philosophy & Economics* 13, no. 2 (2014): 151–64.

Vrousalis, Nicholas. "Exploitation as Domination: A Response to Arneson." *Southern Journal of Philosophy* 54, no. 4 (2016): 527–38.

Walzer, Michael. *Spheres of Justice*. New York: Free Press, 1983.

Walzer, Michael. *Thick and Thin: Moral Argument at Home and Abroad*. Notre Dame, IN: University of Notre Dame Press, 1994.

Weijer, Charles et Emanuel, Ezekiel J. "Protecting Communities in Biomedical Research." *Science* 289, no. 5482 (2000): 1142–4.

Wendler, David. "The Ethics of Clinical Research." *Stanford Encyclopedia of Philosophy*. 2017. https://plato.stanford.edu/entries/clinical-research/.

Wendler, David, and Annette Rid. "In Defense of a Social Value Requirement for Clinical Research." *Bioethics* 31, no. 2 (2017): 77–86.

Wendler, David and Shah, Seema K. "Fair Benefits and Its Critics: Who Is Right?." *Journal of Health Care Law & Policy* 20, no. 1 (2017): 2.

Wenner, Danielle M. "The Social Value of Knowledge and International Clinical Research." *Developing World Bioethics* 15, no. 2 (2015): 76–84.

Wenner, Danielle M. "Against Permitted Exploitation in Developing World Research Agreements." *Developing World Bioethics* 16, no. 1 (2016): 36–44.

Wenner, Danielle M. "The Social Value of Knowledge and the Responsiveness Requirement for International Research." *Bioethics* 31, no. 2 (2017): 97–104.

Wenner, Danielle M. "The Social Value Requirement in Research: From the Transactional to the Basic Structure Model of Stakeholder Obligations." *The Hastings Center Report* 48, no. 6 (2018a): 25–32.

Wenner, Danielle M. "Exploitation and International Clinical Research: The Disconnect Between Goals and Policy." In *The Palgrave Handbook of Philosophy and Public Policy*, edited by D. Boonin, 563–74. Cham, Switzerland: Palgrave Macmillan, 2018b.

Wenner, Danielle M. "Rawls and Social Value in Research: Reply." *The Hastings Center Report* 49, no. 2 (2019): 47.

Wertheimer, Alan. *Exploitation*. Princeton, NJ: Princeton University Press, 1999.

Wertheimer, Alan. "Exploitation in Clinical Research." In *The Oxford Textbook of Clinical Research Ethics*, edited by E. J. Emanuel et al., 201–10. Oxford: Oxford University Press, 2008.

Wertheimer, Alan. *Rethinking the Ethics of Clinical Research: Widening the Lens*. Oxford: Oxford University Press, 2011.

Wertheimer, Alan. "The Obligations of Researchers amidst Injustice or Deprivation." In *Global Justice and Bioethics*, edited by J. Millum and E. J. Emanuel, 279–304. Oxford: Oxford University Press, 2012.

Wertheimer, Alan. "The Social Value Requirement Reconsidered." *Bioethics* 29, no. 5 (2015): 301–8.

Wiedenbrug, Anahi. "What Is Really Owed: Structural Injustice, Responsibility, and Sovereign Debt." PhD thesis, 2018, online available at http://etheses.lse.ac.uk/3793/ [accessed April 3, 2026].

Wilkinson, Martin et Moore, Andrew. "Inducement in Research." *Bioethics* 11, no. 5 (1997): 373–89.

Wilkinson, Stephen. *Bodies for Sale: Ethics and Exploitation in the Human Body Trade*. London: Routledge, 2003.

Wilson, James. "Towards a Normative Framework for Public Health Ethics and Policy." *Public Health Ethics* 2, no. 2 (2009): 184–94.

Wolff, Robert Paul. *In Defense of Anarchism*. Oakland: University of California Press, 1998.

Wolitz, Rebecca, Ezekiel Emanuel, and Seema Shah. "Rethinking the Responsiveness Requirement for International Research." *The Lancet* 374, no. 9692 (2009): 847.

Wollner, Gabriel. "Anonymous Exploitation: Non-Individual, Non-Agential and Structural." *Review of Social Economy* 77, no. 2 (2019): 143–62.

Wood, Allen W. "Exploitation." *Social Philosophy and Policy* 12, no. 2 (1995): 136–58.

World Bank. "Tracking Universal Health Coverage." 2023. https://openknowledge.worldbank.org/bitstreams/021a0fe4-590f-4300-a501-85249d4409a0/download.

World Bank. "June 2025 Update on Global Poverty Lines." 2025. https://www.worldbank.org/en/news/factsheet/2025/06/05/june-2025-update-to-global-poverty-lines.

World Health Organization. "Vaccines and Immunization: Dengue." 2024. https://www.who.int/news/item/15-05-2024-who-prequalifies-new-dengue-vaccine.

World Health Organization (WHO). "Universal Health Coverage." 2025. https://www.who.int/health-topics/universal-health-coverage#tab=tab_1.

World Medical Association. "World Medical Association Declaration of Helsinki. Ethical Principles for Medical Research Involving Human Subjects." *Bulletin of the World Health Organization* 79, no. 4 (1996): 373.

World Medical Association. "World Medical Association Declaration of Helsinki: Ethical Principles for Medical Research Involving Human Subjects." *Bulletin of the World Health Organization* 79, no. 4 (2001): 373–4.

World Medical Association. *World Medical Association Declaration of Helsinki: Ethical Principles for Medical Research Involving Human Subjects. JAMA*, October 2013. https://www.wma.net/wp-content/uploads/2016/11/DoH-Oct2013-JAMA.pdf.

World Trade Organization (WTO), "Declaration on the TRIPS Agreement and Public Health." 2001, available at https://www.wto.org/english/thewto_e/minist_e/min01_e/mindecl_trips_e.htm [accessed January 21, 2026].

World Trage Organization (WTO). "Agreement on Trage-Related Aspects of Intellectual Property Rights (TRIPS)." 2017. Amendment after first agreement concluded on April 15, 1994, online available at https://www.wipo.int/wipolex/en/treaties/details/231 [accessed March 18, 2026].

Young, Iris M. "Five Faces of Oppression." In *Geographic Thought: A Praxis Perspective*, edited by G. L. Henderson and M. Waterstone, 55–71. New York: Routledge, 2009.

Young, Iris M. *Responsibility for Justice*. New York: Oxford University Press, 2011.

Zhang, Li. "Cosmopolitanism and Global Ethics." *Diogenes* 64, no. 1–2 (2017): 15–24.

Zvonareva, Olga, Nora Engel, Eleanor Ross, Ron Berghmans, Ames Dhai, and Anja Krumeich. "Engaging Diverse Social and Cultural Worlds: Perspectives on Benefits in International Clinical Research from South African Communities." *Developing World Bioethics* 15, no. 1 (2015): 8–17.

Zwolinski, Matt. "Structural Exploitation." *Social Philosophy and Policy* 29, no. 1 (2012): 154–79.

Zydus Cadila. "Zydus Cadila Receives Approvals from the DCGI to Start Phase III Clinical Trial of ZyCoV-D—Fully Indigenously Developed Vaccine." Press release, January 3, 2021. https://www.zyduslife.com/public/pdf/pressrelease/Zydus_Cadila_receives_approvals_from_the_DCGI_to_start_Phase_III_Clinical_Trial_of_ZyCoV_D_fully_indigenously_developed_vaccine_-3_1_2021.pdf?utm_source=chatgpt.com.

Index

www.ingramcontent.com/pod-product-compliance
Lightning Source LLC
LaVergne TN
LVHW010948191026
850388LV00003B/23